M000013393

# EVERY DRUNKEN CHEERLEADER...
# WHY *Not* ME?

### Wit, Wisdom and Warmth
### *from your Fertility-Challenged Friend*

by Kristine Ireland Waits

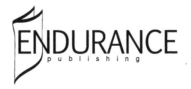

ENDURANCE
publishing

*Books Available at http://www.EnduranceBooks.com*

*EVERY DRUNKEN CHEERLEADER: WHY NOT ME? All rights reserved. No part of this publication may be reproduced, stored in a retrieval system or transmitted in any form or by any means, electronic, mechanical, photocopying, recording or otherwise, without the written permission of Endurance Publishing, Stillwater, Oklahoma, except for in quotations in a review.*

*Copyright © 2010 by Kristine Ireland Waits. ISBN 978-0-615-27406-5. Cover and interior design by Beacon PR led by Stephanie Greenlee. Photography by Madigan E Photography. Printed in the United States of America. Books Available at http://www.EnduranceBooks.com*

*This book is not intended as a substitute for medical advice of physicians. The reader should regularly consult a physician in matters relating to his or her health and fertility.*

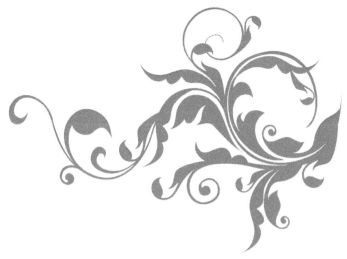

# ACKNOWLEDGEMENTS

Above all I must thank God and my husband. Without each I would not have found the other. And with both God and my husband the trial of infertility was treacherous yet it brought us all closer together.

My battle with fertility challenges ended with great rewards. The making of Sam and Katherine are the subject of this book and the answer to my prayers.

The women in my family are more than the reason I exist. They are the reason I thrive. They can never be thanked enough. I only hope I honored them in the pages to follow.

I must also lift up my best friends and show them to you as a trophy: Laurie Taylor and Nicole Baldwin. Rarely in a woman's life does she find such kinship.

And to my beautiful mother-in-law, Dana Waits, whose passing taught me to love more, to be more and to do more. Thus, in the doing more I have decided to be a writer.

There are several people who helped make the emotional typing of my journal into an actual book. Those people include: Karen Johnson RN, Robert J. Harder M.D., Kim Boatright, Beacon PR and Endurance Publishing.

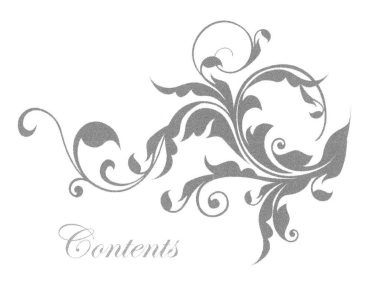

# Contents

Dear Reader ..... 9

Preface ..... 11

The "I" Word ..... 17

Nuggets of Knowledge ..... 23

    Make a Journal ..... 26

    Don't Borrow Trouble ..... 30

    You Are Not Special ..... 32

    Plan Ahead ..... 37

    Control Your Own Care ..... 39

You and Your Medical Professionals ..... 41

You and Your Insurance ..... 51

My Dear Friends, You Need Help ..... 61

Marriage First, Baby Second ..... 79

Morality and Medicine ..... 95

Feel It Up ..... 111

Sarcastic Congratulations to You ..... 117

Waiting is the Worst ..... 133

Melting Your Mask ..... 141

It's Not @#&*ing Fair ..... 147

Prescriptions & Perspectives ..... 153

Epilogue: What Does This Do To Your Book ..... 163

Dear Reader,

I am so sorry you have to read this book, but thrilled you've found a place to turn for information, comfort and a relating story. I am sorry because I know that in order to be attracted to this book, you or someone you know are to the point in a quest to have a family that you feel compelled to seek comfort for a plan that isn't unfolding quite right. You look around and it seems like every drunken cheerleader gets pregnant, so why can't you? You gaze across the restaurant and everyone seems to be pregnant but you. You watch the news and hear of yet another tragic case of child abuse while you long to fill your loving arms with the warmth of a child. I have worn those shoes; gained those same blisters. I can relate to your great need for comfort and understanding.

Beth Moore, a wonderful Bible teacher, often touches on a terrible hardship she had as a child in order to explain how she became the fulfilled, admired woman she is today. She noted in one of her series that many women will come up to her after she speaks and try their best to console her. Beth said that the very best thing she ever heard was from a woman who approached her, took both her hands, looked her deep in the eyes and said "I am so sorry you had to go through that." What a wonderful sense of understanding that sentence communicates. It's far better than long-winded advice or misunderstanding sympathetic eyes. That one sentence is true and honest. It is exactly the way I want to be with you.

No one can know exactly what you are going through. I have traveled my own bumpy road of fertility frustrations with its unique twists and turns. I remember people wanting to do or say the right thing or worse yet, avoid me so that they did not have to do or say anything. So, I would like to redirect the sentiment given to Beth to you as you turn the pages and begin this journey with me: I am so sorry you are going through this.

My Best,

*Kristine*

$\mathcal{I}$ have no official certified authority for writing this book. I am not a doctor, a nurse, a psychiatrist, a psychologist, an infertility specialist or even a phlebotomist. In fact, a few years ago the only acronyms I knew concerning the female body were PMS and BS. The letters DNC, FSH, IUI and IVF (to name a very small few) all sounded like LMNOP to me. So, you can rest assured that this book is not technical or medical, although you will be exposed to some of the basic medical procedures as described from my own personal experience and perspective. While many experts in the field have reviewed and consulted with me on this book, that is only to ensure accuracy and relevance for you. This book is from me, simply a woman who struggled for my family, to you!

My only authority is that I have been there. I know the heartache, the pain, the shame, the feeling of constant questions and no good answers, pretending it's ok in front of your friends and crying in front of the mirror. I know what it is like to smile at your husband and think "he should have married someone who could give him children," while wondering if you ever can. I know what it's like to be in the throes of that thought when you run into his obviously pregnant ex-girlfriend. I have talked to the doctors. I have Googled every related topic; asked friends and experts; and spent countless hours on BabyCenter.com. I have been covered in whelps from shots in my tummy and bottom. I have been covered in zits from the unbelievable amount of hormones they put inside of me. I have carefully placed a pillow under my hiney after sex "just in case." I ate bags of spinach after hearing that it helped somehow. I purchased boxers for my husband (instead of briefs) so that his "boys" could breathe. I prayed. I yelled. I sat in a bubble bath crying. I have been there. I have looked back on my past and wondered if I was getting what I deserved from a less than perfect life; if this was my price to pay for all the bad things I'd done before. I wondered if maybe I hadn't suffered enough to this point, so this was my cross to bear. I questioned whether or not this was some kind of clue that I wouldn't make a good mother, so I'd never get the chance. I know what it feels like for every drunken cheerleader to get pregnant and to ask the question "why not me?"!

Ok, so maybe I don't know exactly what it's like for you. All of our stories and situations are different. But our emotions have some similarities. I deeply needed someone to understand. To talk to. Not to judge me or try to solve my problems. I needed to curl up in the comfort that I was not alone. My prayer is that this book will be that comfort for you. So go get a bag of something chocolate and a pencil to make notes in the margin. Hop in the bath, pull a blanket up next to the fireplace or sit in your favorite reading spot under a tree. This book is all yours. I want you to really feel it. This is my soul reaching out to comfort yours in the way I so dearly needed during my experience. We may have never met, but our shared circumstance makes you a good friend of mine. Let my words take you in their arms and hold you. We share the same tears.

> *It took me:*
> *0 insurance coverage,*
> *1 DNC,*
> *2 rounds of IVF Fertilization,*
> *3 medical doctors,*
> *4 long hard years,*
> *500 options and decisions,*
> *6,000 hours of thinking about my situation and*
> *7,000,000 tears to finally have the family I do today.*

Don't give up.

Your desire to have a family means that you can, in some way, have a family. It may be one of the thousands of medical options that get you there. It may be adoption. It may be a miracle. But you can be a parent if you want to be. And you will have the exact family that God wants you to have. I believe that if I had become pregnant when we had originally started, I would not be the kind of patient mother I am today. I may not have understood the true value of my precious gift. I would not have Sam. He would be another child of another time. And I know that my Sam is the exact person God wants me to raise. Like Garth Brooks sang, "some of God's greatest gifts are unanswered prayers." If you must, roll your eyes as you savor the cliché, cheesy connotation, but it won't make it less true.

Max Lucado wrote a book that's titled *God Loves You Just the Way You Are, But He Wants You To Be Just Like Jesus.* I thought a lot about this while I was nursing my son the other day. He always screams and cries when I stop him from eating to burp him. But I have learned that if he doesn't burp, then he won't get a full feeding – he won't be wholly satisfied. I believe this is why we go through trials in our life. God wants you to experience whole satisfaction. To get there, we need to know the value of that satisfaction. We may think that God is beating us down, when really he is beating our backs to get out the burps. The burps must come before the satisfaction.

It is important that I give a few disclaimers for you to consider as you read this book and share it with others. Here we go.

DISCLAIMER: Don't use my situation as a medical prescription for yourself. In order to understand this book, you are probably going to need to know my fertility situation so I'm sharing that. As you read, please do not take any of this as medical advice but rather listen for some insights and keep learning and growing as you press on.

My situation is my very own. Well, it's mine and my husband's. Our medical problems and the timing associated with our decision making are unique to us. I hesitate in giving the whole truth about our battle because I don't want anyone to use our "formula" or to read this and think "she had a blocked tube and so do I, so I have to do x, y, z like Kristine Waits." Please, please don't do that. Instead, seek out the kernels of truth that you can relate to and rejoice in finding a friend in this book who's been there and cares to support you through your unique circumstance.

DISCLAIMER: This book does have a Christian flair to it, in places. I am a Bible-believing Christian and, when faced with this battle, I turned both to God at times and away from Him at others. I felt it would be a disservice to you to leave my faith out of the story. Without the spiritual warfare, the depth of my infertility struggle would not ring true.

If you are not a Christian and are turned off by "God Stuff" and by those who are Christian, but you also need the support of a person like me, read on! Nothing is so "in your face" that you can't gain amazing insights. The deal is, I became a Christian when I was 21 and had plenty of time to make mistakes that needed forgiving. I don't try to be "holier than thou" or pretend to be something that I'm not. Still, my beliefs largely shaped how I dealt with my situation – the good decisions and the bad, the positive news and the negative, the joyful tears and those shed from great pain.

Upon becoming engaged to Matt, I joined a group of girlfriends I barely knew for a Bible study. My palms were sweating, my heart was pounding and the only thing keeping my car going forward toward its bible study destination was that I thought the girl whose car I was following would think it awfully weird if I spun a Dukes of Hazard u-turn on a 35-mile-an-hour street. So, I went and I learned. And as I learned, it got easier. And that Bible study has since become my umbilical cord to faith. Most of my current friendships were either made in one of those studies or my long-time girlfriends have been in it at one time or another.

So, as you read, please don't roll your eyes at the heartfelt God-related excerpts or the random notation here or there of "my Bible study friend A, B or C." Hang in there for the meat of the matter.

Also, fellow Christians, there are places where you might not like my very worldly tone. My raw emotions from the pit moments of my life thus far are revealed on these pages, often times in the precise words from journal entries I wrote in the exact time of these heart-wrenching days. So, thanks for not judging me and for reading this with a forgiving spirit that's focused on the story and the positive intent as opposed to anything perfect or anything ready for theological scrutiny.

DISCLAIMER: There are multiple entries from my personal journal mixed into these pages. They were written while being hopped up on loads of fertility drugs, some of which made me a little (or a lot) nuts. Without the influence of these medications, I am a much more stable person. You'll hopefully get a feel for that too. Regardless, forgive me if I sound mean or harsh or crazy somewhere. I'm letting it all show and trusting you to gain insight about how you may or may not ever feel and what this journey looked like in my world.

I hope, with my whole heart, that you enjoy!

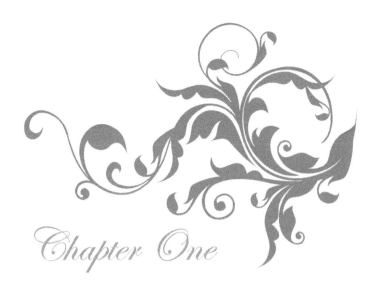

# THE I WORD

*The* thumps of my heart are as loud and fast as a herd of running animals. Is it possible I can feel the slap of their hooves on my lungs? A metallic taste has seeped into in my mouth and my arms have gone limp.

Thank goodness I am in a doctor's office. "Keep smiling," I tell myself.

If I fall to the floor, will the ultrasound technician know what to do?

Only an hour ago had I drummed my fingers on the plastic chairs in the waiting room of my ObGyn office.

Only an hour ago did I carelessly grab at the coffee table littered with magazines and realize I had selected an issue of Parents.

Only an hour ago did I dent my heart as I returned the magazine and make a selection more appropriate for my situation.

Only an hour ago had I been free from the label the word gave me.

The space between then and now followed the path of the sun. My hope rose as I anticipated good news from the doctor that my body had responded to Clomid (Clomiphene Citrate prescribed to enhance fertility). My mood shone as bright as midday as I listened to the physician tell me that my body, habits and lifestyle should be in working order to create a family. Then my mood fell to black and scary as I sat on the table preparing to get an ultrasound.

What had changed? Nothing. I was not different. But there it was, written in pen by the ultrasound technician on the blue and white checkout form, MY blue and white checkout form. I had never seen the word written in penmanship. And I had certainly never seen it associated with me. How could that be my reason for visiting today?

But there it was. Written without thought or concern. Put to paper and then set aside for me until our visit was over.

As the technician turned down the light, I lay my head back for the invasive procedure. Surprised that I can move in this state, I become keenly aware of the tears now dripping past my temple and into my ears.

How could she write that? How could she write that about me?

Emotionally, I was unable to process or accept any more bad news. The Clomid had not worked and yet the pain of that specific disappointment had not yet been felt.

I was fighting against every atom that created my body to maintain composure as I was handed the checkout slip and that big word written in pen. With trembling hands, I reached for the paper taking it as if afraid it would burn me. I now owned the word and was forced to accept it as mine.

The nurse told me to get dressed and to take the form to the front desk. There I could schedule my next appointment. In the same cavalier, carefree manner in which she wrote the word on the paper; on my life, she left the room. Her job was done. I was left alone in a small dimly lit room with the word that forever changed me.

I felt exposed and not from the paper dress. What was I now? A shell of a woman, unable to create and birth a child? Unable to give my husband the beautiful gift of becoming a daddy? Unable to bring a baby into this world and love it with my whole heart the way I so desperately wanted to? My dreams, my prayers, my deepest longings were crashing in on me. A small gasp of air entered my lungs and I was reminded to breathe. I was a failure.

What was the word? What was written as my reason for visiting? What single word could change me? Infertility.

I rarely use the dreaded word "infertility." I may refer to it as "the I word" or "the word" or "fertility-challenged" or a number of other phrases to sidestep that word.

I HATE that I word. I HATE, HATE, HATE that word. It makes me feel like I should give up; like I'm wearing a big sandwich board around my neck screaming "I am infertile." It does not define me! It does not define you! I HATE that word.

I sped from the parking lot of our ObGyn's office into the understanding arms of my best friend. She held me tight and allowed me to sob with moans of pain I didn't know I had.

A few hours later, my husband (Matt) wrote me this email from work: "Hey little buddy. I love you and I hope you are feeling a little better now. I am sorry to hear the news from the doctor today, but I am not devastated by it because I am so happy in our marriage and with our life. I am a little lost for words, but I just want you to know that everything will be ok. First of all, the word infertility just means that, after 12 months of trying, a couple is not pregnant. Secondly, we need to hear from (our ObGyn) more about the current news and what our options are. Maybe there are drugs or procedures that can increase follicle size and egg production. I don't know... but my main point is that we should not be too worried about it at this point or, for that matter, ever. I really do feel extremely lucky just to have YOU. You are all I need. A child would just be a bonus. I love you more than you will ever know. See you in a couple of hours."

So, I caught my breath again and tried to hold on to any thread of hope I could find. I am extremely blessed to have a husband like this. I will get into the husbands topic later. Still, the I word shook up the core of my life. From that point on, I felt defined. I felt deflated. I HATE that word. And I will try desperately not to write it. Yuck.

On the other hand, I have a friend going through a similar situation and she once said to me, "I want to know why some doctors are so scared of the issue, or to say 'infertile' around you." She practically threw her arms in the air like a cartoon character and loudly sang the word. She said, "I know that some people will freak out, but be realistic!" She is practical and direct. She is also a nurse, so she is always frank about medical situations and conditions. I admire her lack of fear about the vocabulary. Maybe you are the kind who can dance to that tune, but I am obviously of the "freak out" category. I know the word is just that – a word. But its undertones do a number to my intestines that I prefer not to experience unless absolutely required.

I'm not sure how authors do this, or even if they commonly refer to their writing process, but I just have to let off one more tiny ounce of steam about the I word before we can move on. Of all the books I have ever read, with the exception of *Oh the Things I Know* by Al Franken, authors rarely share insights into how they write a book that is not about writing. I am going to break the mold.

I didn't start writing this book in some beautiful leather journal with a $400 pen. I don't write tons of scraps of paper and piece them all together (the way I hear J.K. Rowling wrote her fantastic Harry Potter series). I don't have a 1950s model typewriter that is missing the L key. I just use the computer. I do, however, use a keyboard with Bluetooth technology so that there is no cord joining the computer to the tiles I press in order to make the words appear. So, I take my keyboard and sit on the front porch - no monitor to tell me when I have misspelled something, used poor grammar or accidentally hit enter nine times (all of which happen frequently).

The reason for this explanation is that, because I use the computer instead of a medieval form, I had to title the book in order to save the words. And, in a flash of insanity, I saved the initial drafts as "infertility book." See, that word is just far too easy to use. This is not a book about infertility - it is a book about dealing with the difficulties of not being able to conceive. And yet, I still titled the book in such a way. Of all people, I should be sensitive.

It is almost like that word carries some kind of badge. I hate that badge. I would far rather get the "sewing" badge or the "made a mask out of popsicle sticks" badge. I'd even go for another dorky "Hello my name is" badge. I felt like I had to apologize to myself for seeing that word every time I sat down to write.

It is amazing how tainted and dirty that word is for me, for most of us. Yet it is still used on a constant basis when you are in the throes of struggling to have a family. Hesitantly and after a great internal struggle, you decide to discuss treatment with your doctor. The first step is to make an appointment. You look at each digit of the phone number to ensure you have it correct. The kitchen clock ticks loudly as you take far more time to dial this number than usual. As the first ring reaches your ears, you jump a bit, somehow surprised. The second ring and you grip the phone with both hands, ensuring it won't slip now that your hands are sweating. Relieved, you hear the gracious and calming voice of the receptionist. You tell yourself this is going to be alright as she transfers you to scheduling. The nurse answers the phone and asks you the only question she can, "what is your reason for seeing the doctor?" And now you have a choice - to use THE word or not.

We have already talked about that terrible coding sheet when the doctor circles the reason for your visit and under "other", he or she writes... well you guessed it!

A frequent burr in my saddle (I am from Oklahoma, I am entitled to these kinds of phrases) occurred every time I received a phone call from the insurance company. Automatically, I would recognize the number because the display screen on my pretty pink cell phone would announce "call." No name and no phone number were displayed; just that four letter word, call. I grew to know exactly who was calling, even without the name and number. Inevitably, the company would need to urgently discuss my coverage, or the lack there of, concerning an appointment from three months ago that was coded as... the I word. A forceful female voice would declare without concern for my feelings that "we don't cover infertility." They are so cavalier about using that word as if it didn't carry painful weight with its every whisper.

There are also times when you want to investigate the situation more thoroughly in the privacy of your own home so you begin to navigate the Internet. And what do you have to type into the Google box? Yep.

Type it into the "subject" box of major book distributors or other online forms and, from that point on, every time you revisit the site, a whole list of recommendations about assisted procreation pop up. You no longer see recommendations for cooking or the newest Nicholas Sparks love story. Oh no. I wanted to write a letter.

*"Dear Mr. Search Engine,*

*Fertility is not all I am interested in all the time. Give a woman a break for heaven's sake!*

*Sincerely, Kristine"*

There are countless times you will have to sidestep using the word. I hope you can pull out your thesaurus and derive a few wonderful substitutes that do not turn your stomach.

Maybe that big smelly I word would be easier if it really were on a badge so that it would face away from you and make it so that no one would question your situation or behavior.

I am so sorry that you too have to wear that badge. I've been there. Hold out hope.

# Nuggets of Knowledge

*I* am sure that some 84,000 people have given you tips and advice to get you pregnant. I personally feel like the two – tips vs. advice – are different. Tips are actions you are to take in order to achieve pregnancy. Advice is given to help you mentally and emotionally deal with your situation.

No doubt people have given you the tip that you should lose weight, gain weight or eat certain foods, have sex in certain positions, take certain medications... blah, blah, blah. Some of it may be valid and valuable and some of it will be total crap. But the people giving it are doing so because they want to help in your strife to conceive. They love (or at least like) you and want you to have what you want — to procreate. They have either been pregnant and know how to get that way or have seen something recently in the news that is "sure to do the trick." Just take in these informational tips and shelve them next to that bit your mother gave you about your latest haircut. You know, in the "thanks, but I didn't ask for your opinion" file?

I was told by all my friends to stop working out and eat more. They were sure that an extra five to ten pounds would magically put a baby in my belly. Of course I tried that. It didn't work for me. Maybe for a split second I felt good about adding on the weight because, with every candy bar and plate of pasta, I was actively doing something to solve the problem. A troubling part of not being able to get pregnant is waiting without action. You usually have to sit still a full month before you can try another treatment or another avenue. So, with each fork full, I was physically trying something else. Then my period came. Now I was both fatter and just as far away from my maternity goal.

So, this advice section is not going to be one of those try-this-it-is-bound-to-work types. There are plenty of Web sites and Great Aunt Bettys to give you that kind of thing.

Just to compare notes and share a few giggles, here are a some tips I heard or read during my journey.

• Don't have your husband wear "extremely tight shorts." Seriously, if your husband is not Lance Armstrong and he is wearing extremely tight shorts, the problem with fertility might be that your husband likes other men. Sorry to be the one to bear that news.

• No baths a few days after sex in case the sperm are still working their way in there. Oh, now... hygiene doesn't have to go, does it?

• Get body fat in just the right point on the scale. I took this one seriously until I noticed that, at the bottom of the "Fertility Height and Weight Guide," there was a special notice that read, "Note: Height includes 1" heels; weight includes 3 pounds of clothes." Really? Who gives you medical advice while considering 1" heels?

• Thinner women should go on a high calorie fertility diet, which includes lots of meat, fish, pasta, cheese, whole milk and frequent snacks of ice cream, pastry, milk shakes and beer. I did not make this up! It was invented by one Dr. Bates.

• Watch the biorhythmic lunar cycle and have sex only during certain moon phases. Ah, why not try that one?

• There are a thousand supplements and pills. This seems complicated and dangerous considering how they might interact with one another.

- Only participate in certain workouts that are known to maximize fertility such as swimming, dancing, bicycling, moderate aerobics, walking, stretching, tennis and weight lifting. My question is... what does that leave out? Maybe marathon running, but when you are speaking to the general public, do you really need to tell us not to marathon run? Most of us could not and would not do so even if being chased by a man with a gun.

- Acupuncture.

- Eat 2,300 calories per day (that is a ton of calories!) if you have an acceptable body mass index.

- Eat more lean red meat.

- Make an appointment with one of the chiropractors that claim to have fertility boosting adjustments they can make to your body.

- Use the Arbonne cream that my representative swears will boost fertility... as she drives away in her Mercedes.

- Avoid chocolate and other caffeine-rich foods. I laughed out loud at this one. I could no sooner give up oxygen. But I was desperate and actually did try this for about a month. It was torture. And my period came.

- And my favorite – Don't stress about it. AS IF!

Now, that was fun. I am sure you have heard all of those and probably a few other wild ones. Now that those are out of your mind, I just want to give you a few nuggets of knowledge that truly affected me during my plight with pregnancy problems. I do hope these lessons change you in the way they did me. Here they are.

Drum roll please...

**1. Make a journal.**

**2. Don't borrow trouble.**

**3. You are not special.**

**4. Plan ahead.**

**5. Control your own care.**

Tada. That is it.

What do you mean, that didn't change your life?

You want some explanation? (Insert your own audible sarcastic sigh here.) I thought so.

### DISCOVERY #1: MAKE A JOURNAL
### Getting over the fear of writing your thoughts

When I realized I would have to go through more than the average drunken cheerleader under the bleachers on homecoming routine to get pregnant, I confided in a few people including my stepmother, Michele. She suggested I keep a journal. I didn't want the added pressure and stress of something else to do every day, so I didn't think it would really work for me. As it turns out, I thrived on those pages and have continued to recommend the habit to all my friends in similar situations.

I had a palpable fear of someone opening the coveted information (in my case, a Word document) and seeing the depths (that sometimes felt like deaths) of my soul. Somehow someone might uncover things about me that I did not want them to know. I was afraid the nosey reader would know how badly I thought of myself because of my medical problem or think I was shallow for thinking I would be a better mother than some pot smoking hippie or the latest child abuser featured on the evening news. I was terrified to think of the reader's rolling eyes at the grand scale of my pity party.

Then I realized that no one would care enough to take the time to sneak onto my computer and read my thoughts on a daily basis. So, I took solace in my journal as a safe place to let it all out. That journal and the experience of making it was, in large part, the first idea of this book. How ironic is it that something I did, at first, so I wouldn't have to share my story with anyone, later inspired me to do just that?

Sometimes I wrote in this journal as a way to communicate all I have done for the potential benefit of others and sometimes I wrote because it was better to complain to a computer than a person who gets tired of the same old drama. Often I wrote to figure out how I felt. Journaling is for your heart and for the sake of your loved ones.

Writing served many purposes through the years of my struggles with the I word. It gave me a place to rant and scream where no one else could hear. I would turn to my journal when my emotions were so overwhelming that I thought I would either get them all out on paper or they would drown me. A lot of this emotion was hormone induced, but nonetheless real and in need of seeping out from my soul. Those white pages gave me solace when no one else could... or should. They became my haven and allowed me to freely and unapologetically have what my mother lovingly refers to as "diarrhea of the mouth."

Because I wrote these feelings, instead of pouring them onto my husband, Matt, we still have a good marriage. Men are, after all, MEN. They do not communicate the same as women. (Refer to Men are from Mars, Women are from Venus by John Gray, Ph.D. Yes, he may have gotten divorced, but his theories are timeless and relevant.) Matt would have wanted to solve all my problems through rationalization instead of just letting me feel them. My husband is extra-specially wonderful and will let me cry on his lap for no reason, should I need to. Even this hero of a man should not have to referee the scrapping of my innermost tangle of emotions. The poor guy would have gone screaming for the hills in a way that's nothing like the opening scene of The Sound of Music. So, if for no other reason, get a journal for your husband's sake.

Here is a sample of the outpouring of emotions that my journal got to experience instead of my poor hubby.

*Journal Entry*

*After our first In Vitro Fertilization (IVF) did not work. My emotions change every second. One minute I think "it's ok that this did not work, we will do it again and play the odds." The next minute it is "I am devastated, how is this a test of faith when I am proving I have faith... please give us a child." The next it is "maybe I should go back to work and get over it. I'm not meant to be a mom, apparently. I must, somehow, deserve this." I am not sure if any of these are a true depiction of the emotions I have been through. But if you put them in a blender on high for three minutes, then that might be closer to the reality.*

This process also served as a record of my situation. One thing I learned speedy quick about pregnancy issues is that you have to take charge of your own care (tip #5). You may see several specialists and they may all say different things. Or you may stay with one doctor but he will bring up five options at the first visit and only four options at the second. If you have a good record of your discussions, then you can say "hold up pal, what about option #5? Have we abandoned that completely or is that no longer viable and why?" Then write that in your journal too.

If you are like me, when you sit in that doctor's office, you are stressed about being there, trying to reassure your husband that it is ok for him to be at the ObGyn's office and trying to hold back tears while displaying some degree of confidence. Whew. It's exhausting. This is not the ideal emotional state for growing your medical knowledge. But grow you must, and the specialist you are about to see is the best resource. You would not go to your first day of medical school without a way to capture notes, would you?

Our medical professionals and specialists often throw out acronyms and strange, new terms as if they were Halloween candy. If you don't aggressively slow them down and ask them to "spell that," then you will probably miss something important. So, take your journal or at least a yellow legal pad with you into those meetings. Force the doctor to go slow and explain. Work on a time line and get not only the options but his/her recommendation and the reason for those recommendations. Then go home and do some handy research of your own. Detail what you learned through your research in your journal.

Don't feel like you have to be 100% dedicated to it. It overwhelms the novice journal writer. Just write the date at the top and scribble out your situation, feelings, research, doctor's appointment, etc. Then when you are done, put it away. And when you are ready again, write more. The days don't have to be consecutive and what's written is bound by no rules. This journal is made to make you feel better and keep you moving forward – not to give you another action item on your list of things to do. Look at it as an empowering tool in a situation of powerlessness.

I noticed it was much easier to journal when things were going poorly. It became my way of working through the situation, evaluating my true feelings and uncovering a way to deal with them. I have been that way since I was very young. As a preteen and into my high school years, I would write poems to discuss and discover my feelings. It was a very methodical way to map my emotions and true feelings. It usually gave me an ending or some kind of closure. I guess we don't change all that much. Try it and find out if it works for you.

There is a wonderful book called *Modern Girls' Guide to Bible Study*. In the book, Jennifer Hatmaker teaches us how to read the Bible without being intimidated. She writes and thinks very similarly to me - I feel like we are kindred spirits, as I do with all my favorite authors.

Anyway, in her book, Jen writes the following:

*"For you, journaling becomes a written legacy of your conversation with God as He leads you through His Word. It doesn't mean you churn out beautiful prose and poetic revelations. Besides new understanding, authentic journaling includes questions, frustrations, arguments, struggles and doubts – the*

*components of a real relationship. Journaling comes from the same root word as journey. Doesn't that make sense?"*

I agree with what she's saying, but also implore you to journal not only as a record of your conversation with God, as she states, but with yourself, your doctor, your husband, even your great Aunt Betty. Thinking through these things with the care of writing it down or typing it out can lead you to a deeper understanding as you sort through recommendations, ideas, questions and so on. It does not matter how you do this journaling thing, so don't get caught up on that. Just do it in a way that works for you.

## DISCOVERY #2: DON'T BORROW TROUBLE

The fertility clinic we visited was staffed with some amazing women. Both of our fertility specialists were men, but it was these women who made our terrible circumstance manageable. My main contact at the clinic was a wonderful woman named Karen. This nurse was more valuable to me than gold and more precious to me than diamonds. Not only did she offer a wealth of information because she had helped so many women, but her eyes and her spirit seeped compassion and understanding every step of the way. I don't know her outside of the office, but I love what I do know of her warmth in the interactions we shared during some of my most vulnerable moments.

During one of the countless visits when I was getting an invasive ultrasound to check the number and size of my eggs, I began chatting with Karen about some terrible infertility situation I had either read about or heard of through the grapevine. Please note, the grapevine is a terrible place to become educated about the medical profession. I don't recommend it one single bit. Yet, throughout my fertility journey, I seemed to gather the juicy ideas right off the vine. I would research worst case scenarios or causes of infertility. I would discuss with one friend what another friend is going through. I would scare myself to the point of heartburn and headaches.

For about thirty two seconds, I was positive I had cancer or some terrible, debilitating, terminal disease that was causing my inability to conceive. In another instance, I chased crazy medical whims which led me to astronomically expensive herbs that were completely worthless. There was yet another grapevine ripe with the idea that since a friend of a friend had been told by her doctor to take an aspirin once a day - and bingo she got pregnant - I should try that too. No one told me about how dangerous that is and how many bruises I would sustain from even the most delicate touch.

As I shared this cycle of advice and random efforts with Karen, she looked me straight in the face and said "Kristine," long palpable moment of silence, "don't borrow trouble." This hit me like a ton of bricks.

Of course I should not project another's situation, symptoms or results onto my own plate! My plate is full and I am doing all I need to do to get that meal eaten. I don't need to look to the portions of my fellow dining companions. I need to focus on me and what I know about my scenario in order to get to the bottom of it; to make a happy plate, so to speak.

Don't borrow trouble. How simple and yet profound is that? It is like telling someone you want to be a singer only to have them respond "Honey, I love you and I want your dreams to come true, but you have a terrible voice." It hurts for a second, but then you can redirect your actions toward something more viable. When I heard "don't borrow trouble," I thought "well, duh. Don't let your mind dwell on situations that are not your own. Instead, focus your energy on your real issues."

This is not to say you should stop asking serious medical questions of your doctor like, "a friend of mine recently discovered tumors in her uterus that are causing her pregnancy problems. Have we checked for that in me?" The doctor may roll his eyes at you and say that of course he checked that off the list months ago. At least you've asked and have done your part. Definitely ask any question you want to ask. None of them are stupid.

What "don't borrow trouble" meant to me that day was simply "don't take their situations to heart." That's what I want you to consider. If you want to bring up some other ideas or options, do it. That is what being in charge of your own treatment is all about. But don't tie your heart up in it until it is sitting on your plate – or on your already stressful situation.

Don't think to yourself "I have cancer, it must be cancer. Mindy is just like me, we are both healthy and active and seemingly fine and since she turned up with uterine cancer, I definitely have cancer too." Just don't do that to yourself.

Instead, think "I will ask my doctor about this option. Mindy had cancer and I just want to make sure that is crossed off my list. When he tells me I am tumor free, I can move on emotionally and keep my energy focused and my mind as open as possible."

## DISCOVERY #3: YOU ARE NOT SPECIAL

Don't get me wrong, God never has and never will make another you. You are special in that regard. Don't let this lesson ruin your self esteem or anything. But in your quest to be a parent, you are not special. In your frustration at the slow speed of things, you are not special. In your devastation that every friend you have is pregnant and you are not, you are not special.

Yep, that is right. There are zillions of women in this world and most of them want to have babies. It is perceived as our most basic reason for creation and that is even stated in the Bible's book of Genesis. However, according to a recent report from the National Center for Health Statistics, which is under the Center for Disease Control, there were "6.1 million women ages 15-44 with impaired ability to have children." That same list of statistics also reported that there are "9.2 million women who have used infertility services and that 2.1 million couples are infertile." (http://www.cdc.gov/nchs/fastats/fertile.htm) See what I mean - that seems awfully close to a zillion!

When I first began my fight for a family, I remember reading something somewhere about one in ten women suffering from infertility, and suffer we do! Looking back, if I made a list of friends, there would be many more than one in ten with the problem. So, in my world, that is proof that there are tons of us out there.

Follow me for a second...

I am terrified of needles. Well, I was terrified of needles. When I was about four, I faked an injury in the grocery store near the candy isle and continued writhing in pain for several long hours. My mom becoming concerned that I may have done real damage to my tiny limb so she finally took me to the emergency room. The doctor, suspecting my act after responsibly exhausting other diagnostic procedures, suggested they "give me a big shot." Amazingly, I was cured instantly! I shook my 'injured' arm proudly around and announced in a voice that conveyed my surprise "Look mom, I'm all better."

I was terrified of needles, even more so than I was and still am addicted to attention. If there is one thing IVF teaches you, it is that needles are no big deal. However, the first time I had to give myself a shot, I was freaking out.

*Journal Entry*
*Today was the big day. The start of the shots! I carried my huge box of prescriptions and needles to the clinic where they were to take blood and teach me how to use these products. I am not a person that gets nervous in the usual ways like feeling like I am going to puke or pee. Oh no. My nervous stomach insists I go number two. And let me tell you, I parked on the third floor of the garage and could not get to the potty fast enough. Apparently, I was more nervous than I had let myself believe.*

I got through that and marched into the clinic. I was about 15 minutes early and felt very silly sitting in the empty, magazine-filled waiting room with my box looking like a lost, naive, little puppy who was unsuspectingly going to get neutered.

Finally I was taken into a small conference room that had a table full of needles and other terrifying-looking medical tools. Karen talked me through the medication box, asked me if I was overwhelmed and laughed at my nervous jokes (in a good way). We finally got to the part of today's shot. She demonstrated swabbing the top of the vial and then my belly two inches below my belly button and then pretended to stick herself. I thought to myself, "You have got to be kidding me. This lady has probably never given herself a shot before and she is acting like it is no big deal." So after several close tries, sweaty palms, a firmly grasped patch of belly fat and a deep breath, I got that stupid needle in.

As it turns out, it doesn't hurt. In fact I could barely feel it. However, my hands were very shaky, so when I got the needle out, the nurse told me that the raisin-like welt under my skin would not happen every time. She said that when I got the needle in, my hands were shaking so badly I vibrated the needle in and out causing a puff under my skin. The only thing that I felt after that was itching like a mosquito bite.

All of this is to say that Karen, the wonder-nurse, knew I was a big, fat, scaredy cat when it came to needles and she calmly helped me with it. In retrospect, I remember seeing something in her eyes at the time that I couldn't figure out. I understand now that the little twinkle may have been impatience. Not the kind of impatience that you experience when you are in the line at a superstore and the cashier is going as slow as Christmas and you are late for something important like a pedicure appointment. Karen's impatient twinkle was more of a suggestion that I was one in one thousand. They can do it. I can too.

And that is the truth of it. Unfortunately, millions of women have fertility problems and you are no different. See what I mean by "You are not special"? They can do it. You can too.

The ideal aspect to the Lord filling the earth with zillions of fertility-challenged people (and you not being special) is that whatever you are about to experience, it has been experienced before. That is why, for example, love songs work. We all know what it feels like to have a first kiss, to fall in love and to have our heart mistreated. Since we have all experienced it in reality, we can connect and relate with it when George Strait sings about it.

The same is true with regard to the shots I had to take. Uncountable shots in my tummy and then ninety days of shots in my hiney seemed like something I could never handle. (I pray the IVF process has matured past the shots if you have to go that route.) An impossible feat not worth the result - that's what it felt like at first thought, but boy is that wrong!

Anyway, following the twinkle in her eye, Karen told me I was not alone. Just like the women before me made it through the shots, so would the women after me. I too, would make it through. Relish the thought that you are not special. Because of that, you will make it through this process and its physical and emotional pains – just like the rest of us.

This sounds like more of a devaluation of your emotional experience, but that is not the intention. See, if you are not special, then you are a part of a community of others in similar situations and you are not alone. Fertility problems can feel very isolating. You feel like your extremely fertile best friend does not understand your trial regardless of how hard she tries; that your husband is disappointed in you no matter how much he loves you; and that you are stranded on an island alone when, in fact, you are not that special; not that alone.

There are tons of women who are in your shoes and they need you as much as you need them. Even a year after my experience, which has lead to the most perfect son in the world, I still feel the need to talk to my friends going through similar situations because it not only helps them, but it still helps me.

You are only as isolated as you allow yourself to be. If you want to be isolated for a while, go for it. Your emotions are unstable and your ability to communicate is therefore hindered. So, if you feel like taking the easy road and being isolated, then get on with it. But then get over it and realize that you are not special and you are not meant to wallow in your "it's all about me" mode. You are also not meant to be alone, so get over it and get out there.

Nicole, one of my very best friends, also taught me this invaluable lesson after I finished my first unsuccessful round of IVF. I was lying in bed crying and feeling like God hated me (which, of course He does not). She marched over to my house and demanded we go to lunch. "Fine," I said with red face and puffy eyes, "but I am wearing my sweatpants." "You will look cute if I have to dress you myself," was her response.

What Nicole did for me that day was to not let me be special or alone in my battle with the I word. She made me join the rest of the world instead of stewing in my sadness. That sadness was not going to make me pregnant, so Nicole was telling me to get a grip and figure out what to do next.

If you don't have a friend like this, get one. If you can't get one, be one. I am blessed to have multiple friends that I can lean on. Each has their own beauty and each of our relationships has its own history and flavor. Most of the time I am not sure which one I need most at which time, but God has a way of working that out. For example, I needed Nicole to get my butt out of bed and into the real world. And, quite often, I need Laurie for the exact opposite. She is the one I turn to just to melt into a big sloppy puddle on the floor with all emotions raw and uncensored. She is the one whose arms I sought when I read the terrible "infertile" word for the first time. We laugh like kids and cry like preteens together. We pray together and dream together.

I have another friend, Stephanie, who is my support person. She is the one who understands that I take on way too much and is always there to help me. Not just in designing a great invitation to one of our parties, or helping with food preparation (for both I am eternally grateful, especially since it is a request I make of her probably once a month) but she lends support through her words in a way that is difficult to communicate. She knows me so well both professionally and personally that she has learned when to be in the room without speaking and when to sit on the floor with a tea, biscotti, tissues and lots of words.

So, you aren't special. You are one of a million plus women who have, are, or will endure the heart-wrenching battle with the I word and all that comes with it. But, my friend, you ARE special. Your dreams of being a parent are worth dreaming. Your tears for the difficulty are worth crying. This book is worth studying. You may be one of a million, but you're also one in a million. There are things about you that are unique to you; totally special. These things are created in you so you can do something very specifically designed by God for you to do. So, as much as possible, embrace the pain of this journey, face it head on as best you can and take comfort in the fact that lots of other people struggle with this or something else. So, in that, you're not special but, indeed you are irreplaceably special. You need to understand both so that what emerges from this trial is a beautiful triumph.

## DISCOVERY #4: PLAN AHEAD

Like I said at the beginning of the book, I am not a professional in any field of medicine and that includes psychiatry. Therefore, my advice and recommendations in this area are to be taken as you would receive words from a best girlfriend over a cup of coffee. There may be times you think, she is clueless and sometimes you may be right.

Nonetheless, I think we all have to develop our own management style for dealing with the circumstances we'll find ourselves in throughout this struggle. For example: Are you going to tell people you are trying to get pregnant and how? Will you be ready for holidays filled with small children? Are you going to be ok when you get the next baby shower invitation – or go? Can you handle standing in support at a friend's party for their child? Will you be able to handle the moment yet another friend announces her pregnancy? Can you laugh off another comment from a family member asking when YOU'RE having a kiddo?

After much disappointment in myself because of poor responses, I have learned the importance in planning and practicing my reaction and response to those who'll cross my path or, even more importantly, those I love. The best advice I have on this subject is to come up with several 'form' reactions. Prepare yourself before going into a room that contains women of child bearing age. If a situation occurs, pull out the appropriate preconceived reaction and insert it as needed.

These reactions may very well feel like writing with your left hand. You know, it's as if you know you can pull it off but that it will look and feel unnatural and maybe come out a little sloppy. The more your practice your reaction, the more natural it will become.

I won't go into specifics here, because I have given my opinions on how to plan ahead throughout this book. However, without an ounce of depth in explanation, you know I'm right and that this is good advice. You need to think ahead about how you want to handle yourself so that you don't look like a fool, act like a jerk, treat your friends like crap and hurt yourself more.

If you need further help with these kinds of things, there are tons of "real" professional opinions out there. Check out Resolve. They have a great Web site and you can usually find their brochures in the office of your fertility specialist. There is also a Fertility Neighborhood created by Freedom Drug. If you are just entering the fertility challenge, then you may not yet be familiar with Freedom Drug, but they are the pharmacy commonly used to obtain fertility medication. Therefore, they know a thing or two about what is going on. There is also www.babycenter.com whose advice is both written by professionals and laymen. (Note: These companies have not yet paid me a dime to say this. I sure wish they would.) There are also countless books by medical doctors and psychiatrists.

It is not hard to envision scenarios in which you will need a good response. Chances are, you have already encountered three or four last week alone. So, next time you are in the car solo, practice how you will react when someone asks you if you have children, what you will say when an old college friend invites you to a baby shower or when your sister tells you she is pregnant — again.

My dad used to say "remember the five p's: prior planning prevents poor performance." Spare yourself the nightmare and just think through these situations ahead of time.

## DISCOVERY #5: CONTROL YOUR OWN CARE

The importance of taking control of your own medical care cannot possibly be emphasized enough. I feel so strongly about managing your own fertility care that I will come to your house (if you provide the cookies and tea) and tell you in person how VERY important it is to be in charge of yourself.

Before you started reading this specific discovery, you may have been wondering "should I read a section on controlling my own care when I am not sure if I will undergo treatment, and if I do, how far am I willing to go with treatments?" This is what you should be asking yourself! It means you have your head on straight and are thinking logically about an emotional subject. Good for you, girlfriend!

We can explore the question of how far you might want to go with treatment later in the Morality of Medicine chapter. Before you can decide where you stand on the scale of fertility treatments, you need to know that options are available. This book will not tell you your medical options. There are too many and they change too quickly. Instead, I want to teach you how to control your situation so that you are able to make the best and most informed decisions.

You have to flex your big girl muscles, grit your teeth, dig into this issue and control your own care. Ah, its own chapter — the next two actually — because again, this cannot be emphasized enough. To preface these no-nonsense chapters, I must also tell you that there's a spiritual, emotional and moral tie with taking care of yourself. You have tough decisions to make. Just make sure YOU (and your husband) are the ones in control.

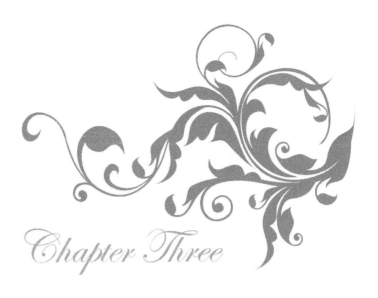

*Chapter Three*

# CONTROL YOUR OWN CARE:
## YOU AND YOUR MEDICAL PROFESSIONAL

*M*y guess is that you started this process in much the same way I did. With an it-won't-take-long attitude and a let's-get-'er-done approach. For us, it started with my annual ObGyn appointment where my doctor and I discussed all that my husband and I had tried in the hopes of a healthy conception. It was a short conversation.

By the way, my regular ObGyn is the world's best doctor - for me. I talk too much and joke even more. I need physicians who can see the difficulty within the comedy. If you are not comfortable with your doctor, get a new one! The ability for you to communicate well with your medical professional could mean success or failure.

After our first visit with the physician, I was left with a slap on the back and a bit of information about a few small fertility-enhancing steps in case we decided we wanted to go down that path. He also offered to write me a prescription for a cheerleading uniform since I had commented that every drunken cheerleader under the bleachers seems to get knocked up on homecoming, and there I sit all financially and emotionally stable with no baby. See what I mean? He's perfect for my personality. I left feeling heard, supported and like I had options to consider. I was on track.

I went home and continued to read massive quantities of books and Internet articles on fertility. I came upon the book *Getting Pregnant: What Couples Need to Know Right Now* by Dr. Niles H. Laurensen and Colette Bouchex. I took a Lifestyle Fertility Quiz, found within the book. I came out with a score of 73. Upon reading the provided Fertility Scorecard, I learned the 73 meant the following.

"50-100 points: Your fertility is likely in good shape, or at least your lifestyle habits are not making significant contributions to future problems. It is also likely you are a well-balanced person who does everything in moderation. If you maintain your current lifestyle, it's likely you will preserve your fertility and your sex life for many years to come."

So with a "don't worry about it" attitude from my doctor and a positive quiz result from that book, I had a renewed sense of hope. As most women know, hope comes and goes with the ebb and flow of... well... your flow.

As time passed and nothing happened, I was extremely disheartened. I decided to communicate my increased concern with my doctor. I found that if I was not doing the talking and the asking, then nothing was getting done. I know. I was told the world didn't revolve completely around me, but I thought maybe it did just a little.

I learned a valuable lesson: no one cares about your desire to have a child more than you do. Likewise, no one knows when your last period was, what problems your mother has had, how long you have been trying, how often you have periods, other medications you take, how often you have sex, or what kind of pains you have in your "down there" better than you do. No one will take better care of yourself than you will. YOU MUST BE IN CHARGE.

You must do research to understand your options involving tests and care. You must keep copious notes in your journal (have you started yours by now?) about what you are experiencing emotionally and physically. Those notes will also remind you that your neighbor Sally told you to eat peanut butter everyday for one month and it will magically make you pregnant. Now that tip may be ridiculous, but one of the small tidbits (though probably not from Sally) may make sense later. If you haven't written it down, you may have forgotten it because you gave someone else control of your care.

You need to understand your body and its condition. You need to understand how the medicines and processes work. You need to understand your insurance. You need to put that negative energy of feeling helpless into positive energy of helping yourself.

Remember fertility treatments are elective. You would not get a breast enhancement without researching options and doctors. Yes, this is somewhat different, but not entirely.

So, how do you know when you have found a good fertility clinic? What are the signs that these folks are legit and completely dedicated to solving your plight? There are several indicators.

The clinic is open on weekends. They are open super early and late into the evening if they need to be. It is difficult to accurately predict when your body will need its treatment. Quite often, your body does not care that it is 6:30 a.m. on a Saturday. Your clinic shouldn't either.

They have medicines, needles and other treatment tools easily available. Unless you live in a major city, fertility medications will need to be purchased over the phone or online and shipped directly to your home. There may come a time when you need to increase your medicine but the UPS man has not yet come calling. A good clinic will be able to "lend" you the goods until yours arrive (at which time you can "pay them back" by giving them the same amount that you borrowed).

A good clinic will be full of spectacular employees. These people will be well versed in their duties and they will not smirk or even think of smirking when you ask them personal and potentially embarrassing questions. They will probably answer your questions before you even ask them. The best clinics may even be so good that they learn your phone number from caller ID and can answer the phone "Hi Kristine, how are you today?" the way mine did.

A clinic dedicated to solving your fertility problem will have endless amounts of information for you to peruse. They will have generic brochures, no doubt. But they will also have packets of information on the treatment you are considering. They may even have classes taught by employees that they recommend or require. They may even sell this book!

A good clinic will not ask you to pay 100% of your fee up front for some procedures that may never come to fruition. Let's say, for example, that you are going to do IVF. There are many steps along the way that may "fail" and thus preclude you from taking the subsequent steps. Therefore, you should not be required to pay for the final step (surgery) before you take your first shot. The good clinic will discuss the financial situation openly and with detail until you feel comfortable.

There are about a thousand other indicators but you will know when you walk in the door if it is the place for you. A woman's intuition is strong, especially when it comes to creating/caring for children. Use yours in this situation.

If you are like me then you probably think the whole world is revolving around your inability to procreate. Alas, it is not. The doctors care about you but they also care that their stats show 59% success instead of 58%. This means they are going to work like hell to help both you and those stat reports. In my heart of hearts, I feel there is a difference between caring about you and caring about their stat results. I am not a doctor, so I don't know for sure, but my guess is that they don't go home to a plate of pork chops and steamed veggies and think "Kristine deserves to be a mother. What more can we possibly do?" Now, they may very well think that. But doctors are people too. They have their own life, family, problems, kids' ballet recitals and college tuitions to manage. They don't have the capacity to think as much about your specific problem as you do – no one does.

So what do you do?

Talk to friends who have been in similar situations. Learn about what tests they took under what circumstances and when. Learn about their medications, experiences and physicians. Get online and research these things. I personally feel there is no better site than www.BabyCenter.com (and, again, they have not yet paid me to say that). Not only does this site have expert opinions, but it also has chats between other women in the community of currently closed wombs. (Note that these chatty women have learned or are learning Lesson #3 of "You're Not Special.")

When you visit the doctor for the first time, tell him/her your complete story. Practice in the car on the way there if you need to. Start with "we have been trying to get pregnant for _____ months/years." Explain what you've tried, your level of eagerness, your amount of stress, your fears concerning both life in general and pregnancy specifically. Bring your husband with you and have him answer the same questions. Bring a list of "could it be this _____" questions if you want to put any fear to rest and get those concerns off your plate.

Here is how the ideal situation should go as you meet with your ObGyn or fertility specialist.

First, you do some research about the doctor before you see him or her, even if this research is talking to other patients. You need to know as much about this person, their education and their theories as you can. Some doctors are general ObGyns and not fertility specialists. You should know the difference before you choose. I have heard about some general ObGyns doing some "more advanced" fertility work than their training affords them. This can be dangerous. I personally feel that a specialist is deemed so for a reason.

Many physicians may have a "give it one more month" philosophy. Of course, you won't find that on a Web site, but you will uncover these kinds of things if you talk to friends and nurses. If this is your regular doctor, then you will already have a feeling for him/her and will have viewed the diplomas and awards in the office. Become familiar with the doctor before your first opportunity to meet.

After your research is done, make both a decision and an appointment. Walk into that appointment with your journal in hand and your medical records from your regular ObGyn (if you are seeing someone new). The more you can get done per appointment, the better. During my first visit to the specialist, he asked the easy question of "when was your last pap." This should be an easy question. Most people don't forget when a stranger put something in her "hoohoo." However, I had been to my ObGyn so many times for fertility enhancement that I had no idea and since I did not have my medical records in tow, we had to call the office and have them faxed over which elongated our waiting time tenfold. So, the better you come equipped, the more you will get accomplished.

Be sure to give the expert your REAL medical history – don't make it up or leave room for question marks and approximations. I learned this from one of those voice-overs on the television sitcom, Grey's Anatomy, which centers around hospital drama. So, while my source may not be credible, it is actually quite smart to make sure your medical professionals know your whole, honest story.

If you are a smoker and are ashamed, tell your doctor anyway. Don't leave out details that you don't think are important. That's the doctor's call. Even if something happened ten years ago to your uterus, it is still significant for your doctor to know. Likewise, lifestyle transitions and other basic habits should be reported with honesty and candidness. If you had an abortion at 16, spill the beans to your doctor. If you struggled with an eating disorder, tell. If you are a kinky, freaky sex kitten – don't tell anyone else in the world – but do tell your doctor. You are not a physician and you don't know what could be relevant.

My ObGyn told me the funniest story. A woman had been coming in for about six months while taking clomid each month. She had been tested and evaluated for everything and there seemed to be no obvious reason she could not get pregnant. This sounds like 95% of the infertility cases I know. At her last appointment she walked in and announced to the doc "I'm not pregnant this month." "Why are you so certain?" he asked. "Our hot tub has been broken," was her response. With a dumbfounded look, he said "and..." "We only have sex in the hot tub," she said embarrassingly. He explained that the temperatures of the hot tub were probably her fertility problem. The couple decided to have room temperature sex and she was pregnant the following month.

So, give your WHOLE history! This story not only underscores the importance of spilling the beans but also shows how necessary it is to have a doctor you feel comfortable communicating with at all times. If this girl had not felt comfortable telling him about the hot tub, she may never have gotten pregnant.

Note: doctor/patient confidentiality is a real bummer. I kept begging my doctor to please tell me who this person is so that, should I ever be invited over for a swim, I can quickly, but kindly, decline. He refused. Ick!

While visiting with your doctor and before taking any medication or undergoing any procedures, you should ask the following:

**Benefits:**
   What is this supposed to do?
**Risks:**
   What are the possible complications?
**Side Effects:**
   How will it make me feel and for how long?
**Alternative treatment options:**
   Why do you want to go down this route instead of the others available?

**Expected Time Line:**

When will we know if it works?

**Expected Outcome:**

How will we know if it works? (ultrasound, new period, etc)

**Managed Expectations:**

If this does not work, what might be the next steps?

When you get home, do some research on your own. If you learned anything in the "journaling" section, you learned the importance of writing down all the information you gathered while at the doctor's office. So, you should be able to query online databases using specific words and phrases the doctor mentioned. This will give you a greater understanding of what to expect and what to ask next time. The World Wide Web can be a scary place of misinformation. So, be careful with your sources. If you don't understand how Wikipedia works, learn!

During the entire process, if you have any questions, call the doctor's nurse for any reason. Obviously, this is the wrong place to call if you want to order Chinese takeout. But other than that, call, call, call. They put notes in your charts, they talk to the doctor, they have the knowledge and they have probably heard the same question already this morning.

I can not reiterate this enough. When asking an ObGyn to review this chapter of the book, he highlighted this with red pen and told me to emphasize this as much as possible. "The nurse is an excellent portal and should be used as much as possible," he said. So, don't feel like you are "that girl" for calling three times a day for a week. I was that girl, for months! This clinic was aware of me and my case because I made it that way. This may make me sound pushy, but I really wasn't. I just had a lot of questions because I did not know a single thing. If you are the same way, then call, call, call. They can't answer questions if you don't ask.

When visiting with your doctor in that exam room, use every moment possible. You will be waiting inside and he will walk up to the door, pull out your chart and look over it to know what he is about to encounter. Then you will talk, he will make notes and finally he will put your file back into the pile. That may be all you get from him. So, make him focus wholeheartedly on you during that time when he is in the room with you. Be inquisitive and prolific so you can wring productivity and progress out of that time together like water out of a sponge. Have a list of questions and feel wholly satisfied in the answers before moving on from one question to the next. Make him really be in the room with you. That 15 to 30 minutes is expensive. Get all it's worth!

Medical care is not something to mess around with. And with this being a voluntary medical treatment, you need to be the one calling the shots. Most ObGyns will give you options and tell you why they recommend what they do. You are the ultimate decision maker. If you need more time, take it. If you want to be more aggressive, do it. This is your experience, your body, your money and your family. Plan the kind of care you deserve and be in that driver's seat.

I have a friend visiting an ObGyn who recently told her "if this does not work, I will refer you to X doctor." My friend has no insurance dictating her healthcare so she can see whomever she wants, whenever she wants. No referral required. Don't get caught up in their lingo or confused by something they say. Ask questions and do your research. You are in charge!

It is terrible to come home after an appointment and feel more disillusioned than when you walked in. The more information you ask for, the more you will get. So, plan to be a little overwhelmed. I have never heard someone say with seriousness "I wish I had less information." You should make yourself fully equipped with the information you need to make a decision, take a break from treatment for a while or hit the gas pedal.

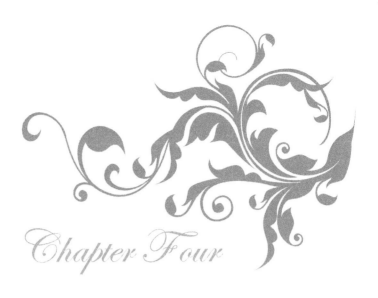

# Chapter Four

# CONTROL YOUR OWN CARE:
## YOU AND YOUR INSURANCE COVERAGE

*I*nsurance discussions are a lot like thong underwear. They leave you feeling uncomfortable, totally exposed and questioning your decision to purchase. So if you arrived at this chapter and thought 'boring, I am going to skip this.' I completely understand. I don't approve, I just know where you are coming from.

But...

That is right, there is a but (just like in thong underwear). You cannot outrun the need to understand your insurance.

Think of it this way. If someone told you "read these few pages and you may get a couple thousand dollars," you would naturally look for your glasses and get ready to read. This chapter is much the same way. You may come across something that will save you some of that hard-earned money. Infertility, or the "cure for infertility," is expensive and usually NOT covered by medical insurance. Be smart.

I had zero coverage for infertility and received zero discounts. I was the first of my friends to go through all of this, so I paved the way with the lessons I learned.

During your first visits to the ObGyn, the most important thing you need to do is explain thoroughly what you have done and what you want to accomplish. The second most important thing you must do is tell the doctor your understanding about what your insurance does and does not cover. This will help you communicate about coverage. For example, tell your M.D. that during your first series of tests, you would like him or her to code the visit not as the I word but as other health screenings, if possible and appropriate.

I have a very good friend who has not had a period for more than a year after getting off the pill. She will make the best mother and she is tired of waiting for her body to work itself out. So, she is moving to a more aggressive gynecologist who is also a fertility specialist. She knows her end goal is to get pregnant and hopefully this doctor does too.

However, when she goes to get tested, the doctor can easily mark the situation down as trying to figure out what is going on with her periods (obviously not the technical term). A woman without periods is like a man without any interest in football; slightly unnatural and a closer look should be taken. This same information will help my friend and the doctor understand why she is having trouble getting pregnant. Therefore, she is getting the needed tests and the insurance will pay for it.

In my friend's case, she really does need to know what the deal is with her periods, regardless of her quest to get pregnant. So, it's not fraudulent, lying or cheating. And if the doctor is not comfortable with marking the designation as something other than the I word, then he or she won't do it. It never hurts to ask and to be aware of who'll be paying for what BEFORE the treatment or testing takes place.

My mother is an insurance woman. She does large business, risk management stuff and not health. But, to the layman, insurance is insurance. I grew up around it as a child and now I pay for it each month. Therefore, this is not my way of advocating cheating the system (or my mother). It is my way of telling you how to work within the system.

Speaking of things that don't hurt to ask, question your doctor about any sort of discounts for those who are not covered by insurance. As before, the very worst he can say is "no" and then you move on and beg some family member for the cash. (kidding... or not.)

I asked my doctor if there were any available discounts and he told me that the majority of his clients do not have insurance that covers fertility enhancements. Therefore, the clinic does not offer discounts because "everyone would be discounted." (Heaven forbid.)

I asked the same thing of Karen, the wonder nurse. (I have an "it never hurts to cover all those bases," mentality and I challenge you to try it.) She told me that the clinic does not offer discounts but they do have payment plans should I need to run that route. She also mentioned that I should speak to the pharmacy because they often reduce the cost for those fertility-less, insurance-less but not hope-less individuals, like me.

I had a situation where my insurance covered, in full, all my lab work. The only stipulation for this is that the work needed to be done at the hospital and not in the doctor's office. Of course I was a novice to my insurance coverage (until now!) and did not have a clue. I just blindly went where the doctor or nurse told me.

During one of our initial visits someone sent me to the lab to give what felt like an entire swimming pool of blood. When I passed the tests, I was happy. When I got the bills, I was not. The lab was connected to the hospital but not a part of the hospital and so I received a big, fat, multi-hundred dollar bill and a notice that my insurance would not cover it. That was quickly followed by another notice, "Oh, by the way this bill is late so we are sending it to collections".

I called my health insurance broker's office and made a new best friend. Kim is dreamy! Seriously, if every insurance company had a

Kim, people would not dread speaking to their insurance company. Her job was to sell my husband's company their insurance and to turn in claims when they came in. Boy, she went above and beyond the call of duty when it came to me.

I told her the situation with the lab work. I am sure my voice was shaky from tears, which were both hormone induced and created out of frustration. A woman not only has to deal with fertility problems but then has to fight with insurance companies as if we needed to feel one ounce smaller. Anyway, she sweetly told me that she would look into it.

That wonderful woman probably made thirty phone calls about this one issue. She called the doctor, called the nurse, called the billing department, called the lab, called the main insurance carrier and more. She was a relentless warrior and she got the job done.

After that situation, I learned my lesson. I got out my insurance policy and I read it cover to cover. Some of it is written in a crazy foreign dialect with sentences that send you from Part II section A to subset C in appendix 7. It is like a treasure map leading nowhere fun. But let me tell you, I was determined to understand my coverage so that I could control my situation. When I got to a crossroads in the literary road, I simply called my insurance angel, Kim, for directions. Now I fully understand where I stand.

Until we get some kind of insurance reform, you have got to do the same. You need to set down that juicy Danielle Steele novel and pick up your insurance policy. In fact, I feel so strongly about this that I recommend you set down this fabulous book and read your policy NOW. Don't worry, I'm not going anywhere and this is important. The next page will help you remember where you were.

Two additional things you'll need as you review that insurance policy: a highlighter (for the obvious reason) and sticky notes. It is hard to remember where the good stuff is in that booklet (that is more like a giant compilation of confusion), so you need some of those neon green and burn-your-retina pink stickies. You will thank yourself later.

Go on, read your policy. Then come back to me.

If you don't have an insurance booklet for the current year that details your coverage, then contact either your employer or the insurance broker to get a crisp, clean, shiny copy.

I was not kidding. READ IT!

I know that may not have been fun reading, but it was no doubt a bit interesting. For example, had you ever before known that part about re-constructive surgery of the healthy breast if you need to get it to match a breast that had cancer? Or had you ever considered the time frame when an adoptive baby is officially covered? Does your policy cover alcohol or mental health treatment? The information in your insurance policy is worthy of knowing and some of it can be down right interesting. However, I hope you're glad to be back together in our little "chat" and that this book is much more whimsical and easy to read!

First things first, you need to seek out your insurance angel. There is someone out there in the insurance world whom you pay monthly. That person should be your spokesperson for insurance coverage. Your local carrier, the guy or gal who sat in front of you explaining (in vague terms) what you were signed up for – that person should be nice. In my case, that was where I found my angel.

However, if you have a hoity-toity carrier who is more concerned with getting new business than managing their current client base, then you need to remember that they are only there to represent a much larger company. Within the structure of this enormous insurance maze, there is bound to be one person who will take you in, return your calls, answer your questions and be a "real" person to champion your cause.

Once you find your insurance angel, do something wonderful for her like sending a personal note, box of chocolates, photo of you smiling. Another idea might be to send a note to their boss telling him that she deserves a raise. Let's face it, she probably does deserve a raise for what she is about to do for you!

Dealing with insurance was the most emotionally crippling part of the battle for me. My pulse quickens as I remember seeing calls on my cell phone that would say "unknown" on the caller id. I knew I would be asked again to explain in detail the situation - my private heartbreaking situation. Corporate people and insurance representatives are dealing with the most personal of issues but are most often set up to be very impersonal.

 I remember the disappointment when I would go to the mail expecting a birthday card and instead receiving a letter from the insurance company. Most of the mail would be an explanation of benefits (E.O.B. for those in-the-know) that either does not explain much or explains so much that you are told to both pay a bill and not pay a bill. I wanted to cry and pull my hair out. So, being a bald, puffy-eyed girl, I began to avoid the situation by not dealing with the calls. This is not an action I recommend. It only serves to escalate the problem. (Ever see the movie House of Sand and Fog?)

I will admit being impersonal truly is the only way insurance companies can accomplish the management of thousands of people and their medical situations. I don't deny it is (most of the time) relatively effective. I just don't personally have to like it.

Make sure when calling these insurance companies that you get the name, number and extension of the person with whom you are speaking. Of course, I recommend putting that in your journal. It is better than writing it on one of the hundred sticky notes you have posted in unheard of locations never to be seen again.

Eventually I learned not to worry about those calls. What you need to do is picture the people behind the impersonal madness at a Jimmy Buffet-like BBQ, wearing Bermuda shorts and maybe a big hat adorned with a brightly colored parrot. They are all regular folks just looking for a paycheck. And chances are, they are nicer than they originally let on. You must find the people behind the phone call if you are ever going to get something done.

I began my journey through the insurance maze like a frightened child: naive and in need of a caretaker. I ended with a sense of control. This is not to say that things were covered under my "coverage." In fact, 90+% of my care was not covered. However, I was able to identify areas that might be covered and I was willing to fight for what potentially could be covered. I was also aware of what would never be covered and could come up with a plan for if, how and when I could still make it all work.

You must become empowered by becoming educated. Knowledge is power!

*Chapter Five*

# My Dear Friends, You Need Help

*Y*ou now know my top five pieces of advice for those of us in this "pregnot" situation: make a journal, don't borrow trouble, you are not special, plan ahead and control your own care. I hope you feel inspired, encouraged and armed with a new sense of purpose. But, let's face it. Our friends are in need of some work also.

Most people don't know how to deal with friends who are having fertility problems. So there will be a lot of mishaps. It may take you years to have children and your friends, who are there for you, will have troubles and trials of their own during that time. They will need you. While you are still fighting for your family and hurting, muster the energy to care about your friends too. Friendship is a give and take. True friends of the fertility challenged will give a lot but also need to take sometimes.

If you are fertility-challenged, then ear mark this chapter and pass this book to your girlfriends. Or better yet, buy them their own books and bookmark this page! If you are a friend to the fertility impaired, then grab your highlighter. You may be the best friend in the world, but this is a tricky time for all of us and I am sure you will want to preserve as much friendship as possible while being the best kind of friend you can possibly be.

This chapter was created after multiple requests from others who said things like "I don't know what to say," "I didn't know how to respond when…," "I don't know anything about these treatments or procedures and I want to show I care. This is just such a big learning curve, not to mention an emotional roller coaster."

There is no doubt that we, the fertility challenged, need you, our friends, right now in the heat of these life changing, heart breaking moments. Thanks for taking time to understand the situation a little better. Read on for insights and kernels of wisdom but don't stiffen up as if this is a checklist you must always remember. Friendship has its ebbs and flows and a level of forgiveness. Care and be real. Be sensitive. Be unselfish. Allow your friend to care about you and be real too. Beyond that basic premise, maybe some of these insights will resound with you when the time is right.

If you're like those requesting this chapter, I am sure you are asking yourself the following questions.

*How can I help?*
*What should I do?*
*What shouldn't I do?*
*When and what should I ask about?*
*How can I best support my friend during this?*

These are wonderful questions. If you are the kind of friend who picked up this book in order to have even one of these questions answered, then you are already worthy of a gold star. Most people are so concentrated on their own life that they seldom stop to care so much about another. You are a wonderful friend and the gesture of reading this is HUGE to us! Please let your friend of questionable procreation know how much you care and what you are doing.

If you are a woman, you know you are difficult to understand. If you are a man, you should know that we women know we are complicated creatures. In a personal, hormone overloaded, tricky situation like this, we never know the right thing to say or do and our tense disposition sends everyone around us into anxiety about how to behave in our presence.

The truth is, some of the time we know what we need from you and some of the time we have no idea. It is your constant and unwavering friendship that will get us through this, even if you do it wrong and we mess up too. Here is an insight entered in my journal a few months after our first IVF procedure did not work.

*Journal Entry*

*It is funny the way women are. It is like I am trying to comfort all of my friends through this in order to comfort myself. My Bible study group shows their sympathy with droopy-eyed looks and whispers about how it is so unfair. Then I tell them I am fine, implore them not to worry and reassure them that I know God is with the situation. (The latter of which I strongly believe.) I tell them what wonderful people they are and what a blessing they are in my life and in others'. I build them up when what I really need to do is personally break down. I guess that is just my way of coping; my way of getting to tomorrow; my way of not losing myself and my friends in this, my time of greatest trial. Maybe if two people are leaning on you, then they are actually holding you up.*

The following recommendations may not ring true for all women. We are, after all, unique. However, a large majority of would-be baby makers on the planet would likely agree with me that the following tips are separated into three main categories: General Rules, How to Talk and Fat Mistakes. Those of you who are more socially awkward than the average high school tuba player might want to read the Fat Mistakes section first, in order to preserve any further wrongdoing.

There should probably be a Social Bill of Rights for those of us in this situation. I picture it being read either with one hand held over your heart like the pledge of allegiance or with one hand on the bible as a trial witness is asked to do. It would probably start like this: We, the fertility challenged people of the universe, in order to form a more perfect living environment… However, I'll spare you the clever quirks mixed with lawyer's jargon and keep this in simple advice & story format.

To uncover this advice, I did some completely unscientific research. I asked the multitude of my girlfriends who are going through similar situations what tips their friends need, what blunders they have been privy to and what has helped them most. I also asked their best friends what they wished they knew about how to help.

You should know that "be sensitive" was the top advice bit I got from those of us who've been in the struggle. Likewise, the top question I got from friends was "what should I say?" Here's a summary you can learn from and relate to.

## GENERAL RULES

**Please start listening to us.**

When we come to you with our news that the cards of our fertility are a part of a hand that should be folded, you don't need to say anything. Just take a large sigh, let your eyes fill up with tears on our behalf but don't feel obligated to make excuses like "it will happen" or to stroke our head with proverbial encouragement. More often than not, we need someone to recognize our breaking heart, not to sew it back together.

In the midst of doctors, procedures and decisions, a woman can feel unheard. It is a much-needed refreshment to have you there to hear us.

When we call you, if you will just listen to us, you will solve ninety percent of our worries. If you don't say much, then you are less likely to say something wrong. Now there will be days we want to talk and days we want to be comforted, so your lack of talking on comfort-needed days may seem insensitive. Even so, just listen to us and you will know which day is a just listen day and which is a please talk back day. The rhythm of our friendship and our history will be the guide so don't worry but, when in doubt, just listen instead of advising or trying to over-encourage.

**Don't leave things open ended.**

If you say that you are there if we need you, then be there a lot. We need you a lot. Call us, check in on us, ask us questions, stop by, invite us out. It is kind of like telling someone "we should have lunch sometime" and then not following up with a date. There are plenty of partial friends out there. If you want to be a real friend, then please show some follow through. We need you in a way that is hard to communicate. You might be the one that makes our day ten times better.

*Journal Entry*
 *The commercials about depression always ask if you have stopped being interested in your favorite things. And I have. I don't know if I would accept the help if someone offered it to me. I get offers like "call me if you need to talk" or "I understand what you are going through" or "I am here if you need me." Let me tell you if someone really, really needs you, they don't know how to ask or how to say what they need. They also don't want fraud-like "understanding". In fact, I appreciate when people don't know. I get to explain in detail and, in doing so, can often figure myself out more. But please, please, please don't compare your life to mine or just because someone else you know went through this means we should get together over coffee and become well.*

**Be aware.**

If we are together and someone just announced her pregnancy, it's ok for you to slightly give us that knowing look. That understanding glance may be the one thing that alleviates the embarrassing tears. Please make sure that look is not one of "poor you." You know that gesture. It is the one where you lower your head, furrow your brow and make droopy eyes. It should be more a look of "are you ok, 'cause if not, I will fake a seizure right here to get the attention onto something else." This gesture is more of a very light motion of your head up with a tiny squint of mischief in your eye. If you give us the "poor you" and not the "seizure ready" look, then it will be you that makes us cry and not the new news. Tricky, we know. Sincerity and the depth of our friendship will be the two factors that make this succeed or fail. **Save us.**

If we are in a room with other moms and the only subject is pregnancy, child birth and/or children, then please change the subject if only for a while, for our sake. There are 84,000 other topics in the universe that can be discussed among friends. Just pick one and go for it. Tell an embarrassing story about yourself. Discuss the newest movie featuring some super hot actor or extremely talented person. Usually this can be good for a 20-minute conversation which will give us the emotional break from having nothing to contribute due to not yet being a mom or being pregnant. Talk politics if you must. Just be our savior when it comes to the direction of the conversation. Chances are, even if a woman is not undergoing fertility treatments and has chosen, for whatever reason, not to have kids yet, that they would rather not discuss your kids' bowel movements or the tee-hee funny (to you) thing your kiddo said at breakfast.

**Be sensitive.**

Be sensitive to our feelings about what is going on. This is a general rule because it is so very, very general. Being sensitive is hard to quantify with examples. However, a resounding remark from my friends in this situation is "just try to be as sensitive to our sensitivity as possible – without being overly sensitive." Oh, you're a woman. You get it. CARE.

**Be extra sensitive on baby shower days.**

If we are trying for a baby and have not conceived after nine months or so, we would appreciate it if you would recognize how difficult it is for us to attend or host a baby shower. Truth be told, we would prefer it if we weren't even allowed to attend them! But that is a dream world.

All sarcasm aside, it's heartbreaking for us if you don't invite us. It's heartbreaking for us if you do. We are friends and we want to support you if we are emotionally stable enough. So, invite us but don't follow up for the RSVP or put us in a place to explain our awkward blah about the occasion. Depending on the person having the shower and the state we're in with our own infertility journey, showers may not be a big deal. However, if we're right in the midst of the rut where we can barely catch our breath due to our own personal grief, being expected to host or attend something cheery is sheer torture. Just let us take it one day at a time and allow us to decide in the ten minutes before the shindig if we will be there. This is a leniency we desperately need.

**Screen the news.**

Don't assume that we are ok with hearing so-and-so is pregnant or so-and-so just had her baby. Ask us, when you find out about our situation, how we want to talk about this kind of stuff. Use good judgment and understand we will probably change our mind a few hundred times. If we are having a sad day, then maybe tell us "Jenny is pregnant again" at another time. Or, if we are feeling optimistic and happy, then give us the news in a frank way. Don't give us those puppy dog eyes which ask us to tell you how crappy it makes us feel. Just tell us and then move on. If we want to discuss more, we will start that conversation.

Regardless of circumstance, we eventually need to know if so-and-so is pregnant or had her baby. We are trying our hardest to hold on to friendships while keeping our emotional composure. So, if you know someone is pregnant, then tell us before that person does. This gives us time to prepare. Please, please don't tell us in large group surroundings. If you just learned of a pregnancy and the pregnant one is about to blow the news to the whole group, then take us on one of the "required to go in twos" restroom breaks and tell us first. This will save a potential blunder of cascading public tears of jealousy.

**Know your audience.**

Create a "politically correct" ending to your story if you are telling a group it took you a whole six months to get pregnant. Not only is this helpful for those of us you know are already going through fertility treatments, but it's good for general less-known groups too. How can you know another person's sensitivity if you just met? If you don't know their situation, they may be having fertility problems and that six months sounds like a slap in the face compared to their four years. So, if you are talking about how it seems oh-so-long to wait to get pregnant, then end with: "I just hate it for the women who have to wait so much longer. It has to just be terrible for them." I personally had a friend who sent out a mass email about her pregnancy. She told us it took her a whole two months of trying and mentioned how difficult the waiting was. I wanted to vomit.

**Allow us to leave.**

We would appreciate permission to leave any party or social gathering early and without an excuse. As one of our very best friends, you should automatically know it is because we got sad and needed the comfort of our couch and that it is perfectly fine. Don't go after us or make a scene about it. Let us go. If we need you, we will signal you in some way. But, don't point it out to others or make an issue of it later. There are thousands of little things, along with the big ones, that may cause us to need to get away. Just understand that and let us go.

*\*\*Starting to feel like this is a set of rules? Remember, you're reading for insights that could come to mind later as the time is right. If you care about your friend and have a history of love and loyalty together, much of this will work out! Keep your chin up and read on. Thanks for caring about your friend enough to read this. Don't walk on egg shells.*

*You can break all of these little guidelines and still be ok if you're genuinely coming from the best motives. Just take this for what it's worth.\*\**

**Distance is ok... sometimes.**

Distance is a tricky one. There will be times we don't want to talk, so we won't answer the phone. There will be other times we want you all up in our business. The best way to do this is to use your friendship radar and read us the best way you can. Just don't judge us too harshly. We know this is hard on you and you know this is terrible on us. Please just stand by us and do the very best you can. If you're confused, leave a voice message saying: "I feel like you're wanting some space, so enjoy that! Have a chocolate shake on me. Call me when you can. I care about you – miss you. I'm dropping by on Friday if I don't hear from you before then, ok? Love you, bye!" Keep things lighthearted but call us out on the issue if you need to, it helps us know you care.

**Note to the One in Need.**

If you're in the throes of your fight for a family, you are probably being a bit difficult right now. Hopefully, your friends understand. Just remember to give them a little break and tell them what you want from them. If you need to talk, then talk. If you need to be silent, then when they call, tell them the truth. Help them understand what you want from them. It will make it easier on you both.

## HOW TO TALK

During the research, a friend of a fertility challenged woman asked me:

"I don't like to pry, but I don't want to come off inconsiderate or like I'm not thinking about her either. At what point is it ok to ask about results from a procedure or doctor's visit OR is it never ok to ask and better to wait until you are told?"

This is a fantastic question, don't you think? This is a woman who really wants to be there for her friend but does not want to upset her or overstep any imaginary bounds. I applaud her friendship loyalty and her concern about being sensitive.

Most women will, of course, be different. So there is no blanket answer to the posed question. However, there is a basic rule you can use that will help. If your friend has told you about the test, then she wants you to know. If she told you the time and date of a test, then she wants (and probably needs) your serious support. So, if the appointment is at 1 p.m. and she calls you to "check in" at 3:15 p.m., then the first thing you should do is ask about the results, how she feels and what comes next. However, if she has not called you by say 6:30 that night, then it may have been bad news and she needs some time. Call her first thing in the morning and tell her how much you have been thinking about her and then ask for the scoop. This will have given her the much needed time to process whatever's happened, but it also lets her know how very much you want to join her in the battle.

The following are a few additional tips on how to talk to us. I hope they aid, even a tiny bit, in helping you communicate with your buddy.

**I beg of you, stop saying "it will happen."**

This is the number one thing that we are all extremely tired of hearing. Somewhere, subconsciously, we know it will happen but it hasn't yet and those words are only empty promises. They are promises that YOU can't make. The underlying truth, which every woman knows even if shortsighted at the present time, is that if we want to be a mother, it will happen one day. Since it hasn't yet, we feel cheated and reminding us "it will happen" only invites our heart to dwell on the fact that it hasn't yet. So just lose it from your vocabulary.

**No one can advise you better on how to be a friend than the friend herself.**

Non-verbal cues often speak louder than words. Listen to your friend and watch her reaction to what's going on around you. That will tell you best how she is doing and what she needs.

**Don't tell us to "give it time."**

This will make a friend/relative/spouse pull hair out. We have been giving it time! We don't consider ourselves to be in this situation until we have given it more than ample time. Probably, to your ears saying "give it time", sounds like "I don't want you to be upset. Surely something will happen for you. You deserve to be a mother. Just give it a bit more time." But this is not at all what we hear. Consider replacing "give it time" with "let's go get some tacos." Personally, tacos solve a lot of my problems. Your friend may want chocolate or vodka instead, but you get the drift.

My husband loves to toss out the adage "rub some dirt on it" when I'm only slightly hurt (emotionally or physically). It's his very male way of telling me to get over it. He used to tell me "it's a long way from your heart," meaning "you are not going to die from whatever it is that is ailing you, so enough already." However, he has since learned that, since I am all female, everything in the world is "close to my heart."

Anyway, his "rub some dirt on it" insensitivity is very similar in nature to our dear friends telling us to "give it time." It makes us feel like you are not validating our struggle. It feels like your flippant attempt to brush us off, as if you want to rush our concern and move on with the conversation. You might feel that, in another month or week, we will be just fine but in that moment, our world is crashing in and you being careless is just another blow. We are hypersensitive about everything if we've started hormone treatments so watch out! Logic may be taking a far back seat to our own dramatic perception of reality.

**Be frank.**

A girlfriend told me a great story the other day. She had gone to a baby shower (probably her 84,000th one to attend). Upon watching another expectant mother opening another package of adorable pink or blue teensy booties, her pregnant friend turns to her and quietly says, "I bet this sucks for you." When I heard of this, I wanted to call this wise little mama-to-be and give her a gold star. Why? Because of course it sucked for the fertility-less one. She was elated for her round bellied friend but she felt entitled to be in the same condition! She felt robbed of something wonderful and beautiful and precious. She felt robbed of this wonderful baby shower experience. Yes, it sucked for her and it was a moment of relief to be cared about, heard, related to and loved in the midst of everything else.

Oftentimes friends and family are afraid to talk to us about fertility dilemmas. They think they might say something that will upset us or turn our happy mood upside down. For most personality types, true friends appreciate frank talk. Yes, just frankly talk about it. It gives us a safe place to share the emotion and to download our feelings. It gives us permission and a big cushy welcome mat to work through it out loud.

*Journal Entry*
> *I have tried to have a private battle before. Something I would keep only to myself about myself. I have never been able to. I have wonderful friends and family that are always in my business. Sometimes this may feel like an intrusion but it is such a gift as I am never allowed to sulk and must share my innermost hardships because sharing forces you to give it, if only for a while, to someone else.*

Being frank should also be noted in the general rules section when it comes to telling us someone is pregnant. We are not nearly as breakable as we may be letting on. Let us know what we need to know and let us know that you get us. That is it.

**Allow us to talk about ourselves and our situation (at length with no reservations or limitations).**

Please understand that we want kids just as much as you've ever wanted anything in all your life. It's all-consuming. There is a lot on our mind and even more in our heart. Allow us to get those things off our chest. We need this outlet so badly. It may be the most precious gift you can grant us on this journey.

**Ask us how we are doing with everything.**

If we don't want to talk about it, we will tell you that. The fact that you ask is wonderful. It lets us know that we can come and talk to you when we are ready.

**The same friend that asked the question of "when to ask about results" also asked "is saying something as simple as 'I'm so sorry' hurtful? Does it come across as not caring?"**

Absolutely not! Unfortunately, you can't make it better. You can't put a baby in our tummy and therefore kind words are all you have. Telling us "I'm so sorry" or "I am so sorry you have to go through this" is a great response. For the closest friends, add in an "I love you" and a hug and you will have really done all you can.

**How to Talk Note to the Friend in Need:**

Surprisingly, our friends need to hear from us as much as we need to hear from them. Friendship requires care for another person and any true friend will be dying to do what they can to comfort us. We will find that we will have to forgive them along the way.

## FAT MISTAKES

The best way to highlight the big fat mistakes is to give examples. No animals were harmed during the making of this section, though feelings were.

**Instead of comparing, try just caring.**

Stop comparing us to others in an insensitive way. It is nice to hear that there are others out there experiencing similar hardships. It makes us feel less isolated. However, if you are not the person with this problem, then you don't need to compare our stories. It feels faked almost as if you are trying to give us advice in a weird third-party way. Don't compare us to your other friend(s). Just listen to us and care. That is what we need most.

*Journal Entry*
> *Today I told a friend to please not compare my situation to others or to trivialize it by comparing it to when she could not get pregnant for a few months. She felt terrible. And I spent the rest of the day making her feel better. I had to convince her that she was a good friend and that she need not be so sad about her rudeness. What a bunch of freaking crap! I am the one in need here. Please see this!*

**We're trying our hardest to be normal– give us some room.**

Please allow us to have blood shot eyes at a baby shower, child's birthday party or the announcement of a pregnancy without being questioned. Those eyes are allowed to be a result of either crying on the ride over or having a shot or two of tequila.

I was at a baby shower when another friend announced her pregnancy. I melted into the background and went to the restroom while the newly pregnant friend was congratulated. I had planned to sneak out of the event, without being noticed, but a big mouthed friend had other plans. When I came back into the room, she asked loudly "are you ok?". I was mortified. The attention of the entire room came my direction. I was embarrassed and ashamed.

**Think before you speak.**

No one, under any circumstance, should follow the response of "no, we don't have children" with a response like "what's your problem, don't you like kids?" That person may have fertility problems and you are just a big fat idiot. This really did happen to Matt and me. I could have clobbered that creep. Obviously, this doesn't happen if you're a close friend of someone experiencing difficulty, but it's good to keep in mind for other public occasions and for protecting your friend from similar idiotic comments.

**Shut up about your kids for a while.**

This sounds hostile and it is not intended to be. If we are friends, then we love those kids of yours. I pray that goes without saying. It is just that we need to think about something else every once in a while. Chatting constantly about pregnancy and kids for hours on end is a general rule but since this is such a big one, it needs to be noted here too.

I have a friend who went on a weekend trip with a few other couples and the women talked about their pregnancy, other's pregnancies, birth, infants, toddlers and all other similar topics for four hours straight! No exaggeration – four hours! She was miserable. A couple of the women even knew that my friend and her husband were experiencing difficulty. After hearing that story and being a friend-in-the-know, I wanted to hit those girls in the head with a dirty wet fish. People really need to be more considerate.

**Note to the Friend in Need:**

If you can think of more of these blunders, then send them to me and I'll either post them on a Web site or make a supplementary book for others to gain awareness (and a few good laughs). I bet there are some doozies out there.

I have been both the friend in need and the friend needing to help, so I know how difficult the situations can be. And, I would like to say that writing this book does not make me mistake-less. You would think that while concentrating vigilantly on the blunders I have experienced, I would be at the top of my game in stopping those similar "accidents" from happening to my friends that are currently in need. However, I recently blundered in a big way.

During Labor Day each year, Matt and his two best friends head to Kansas to kill their fair share of dove. So, this annual occasion has become aptly named "The Dove Massacre." This is a male bonding time to which no woman should ever be subjected. In fact, one of the friends is experiencing fertility problems and, upon arriving home from the Massacre, I asked Matt if they discussed it at all. His response was that the friend had just said that "it sucks." "Did he elaborate? How is she feeling? What is their next step? Who is their doctor?" The questions poured out of me. Matt just looked at me like a deer in headlights and said "He just said it sucks." I will never understand how that is enough for men!

Anyway, after the Massacre, we host the Dove Feast during the Oklahoma State University Football Homecoming weekend each year. We invite all our friends and coworkers for the party. After so many years of this event, we have mastered the dove recipe and I can honestly say it is a big hit! This year was no exception.

Friends started arriving and, as usual, the men went to the back porch to grunt, guzzle, belch and scratch things and the gals began to congregate in the kitchen around the chips, cookies and casseroles. It did not occur to me until one of my fertility challenged friends walked in that she had stumbled upon an entire kitchen filled entirely with pregnant women. There were five of us hording the artichoke dip with round bellies.

I should have thought ahead. She is always early to parties and so I should have made sure this kind of shock would not happen. I should have told her in advance that there would be several pregnant women at the party or I should have somehow lessened the blow. Maybe there was nothing I could do, but the fact that I did not even realize what was going on until it was in the throes of happening was terribly insensitive of me.

I remember being that girl. I remember seeing everyone with the "glow" and feeling like I wanted to run away. Sometimes there is nothing you can do and sometimes there is nothing you should do EXCEPT be aware. I was not aware of the situation and the circumstances from her perspective and I should've been. See? That is the first step and everyone gets it wrong sometime. Hopefully by thinking this through and concentrating on this as you read, it'll make a difference for a friend the next time around.

Anyway, when I realized the situation and found a moment alone with my uncomfortably un-pregnant friend, I apologized. She told me that it did "suck" (as the men so eloquently put it) to walk into that room but she reminded me that we are all friends and so there was nothing to do. I could tell the rest of the party was difficult for her. Acknowledging the situation won't make it go away but it will let your friend know that you understand and care.

The very best advice to both the friend in need and the friend needing to help is to be the kind of friend you would like to have. You were selected as a friend in this life and a confidant in this circumstance for a reason. You get us and we need you.

# Chapter Six

# MARRIAGE FIRST. BABY SECOND.

Allow me to share my perspective on marriage and men so you can pick and choose what is most appropriate for your circumstance. Regardless of where you are in your family quest, making the most of your marriage must come first. It is never too late to strengthen a marriage. Every marriage, be it blissful or battered, can use strengthening.

Take advantage of right now and, if you haven't already done some of the following recommendations, then use this chapter as a way to inspire you to make the most of the childless moment for the enrichment of your marriage. Talk with your spouse about the treatments you've done or wish you had done. Exploring this as a couple may unfold a personalized plan of action and unimaginable comfort and hope both in your marriage and as you face the difficulties and decisions that accompany fertility challenges.

I am not a marriage expert by any stretch of the imagination but I have a pretty good one... marriage that is. I truly believe the reason for that is work. We have worked on this relationship. We have worked on our own development so we can have a stronger marriage. We have prayed.

We have studied. We have read. We have cried. We have laughed. We have shared.

I want to encourage you to have the best marriage you can as you enter this trying time of fertility complications. All relationships will be tested as you suffer through this battle, but none as much as your marriage.

 We are always told that couples fight most about money and sex. The way I figure it, fertility problems include both. So you best be prepared.

Here is an excerpt from my journal that shows just a brief few of the male inadequacies that might pop up during the fertility-less stint:

*Journal Entry*
> *We first had to go through a class via the fertility clinic. I think I forgot to mention that both our doctor and the clinic are in a larger city, about an hour from our home. This was a husband and wife class to inform us of the process, medications, risks, science and requirements both physically and financially. It was a time for some of our questions to be answered. There were ten other couples in this class. It was interesting to watch the interactions, or lack thereof, of the people in this class. Being only 26, I was by far the youngest. And Matt, being 27, was the most interactive of the male bunch.*

The man on my immediate left, obviously a cop because he carried a gun, fell asleep several times and was awakened with quite a head jerk reaction. A man across the U-shaped table took two or three phone calls during the course of the two-hour class. With all of the emotional and physical pain his wife is planning on going through, you would think this jerk could leave the phone in the car for an hour. And, of course, there was a know-it-all couple at the bottom of the U. He would interject things like "Master Card gives you 2% back so you should put your procedure on the card." Great, did they pay for that inadvertent commercial? Is that how they are financing this deal?

You can sense my unsympathetic, sarcastic tone which was probably doled out on great guys who at least were PRESENT; a sign of my time of life I suppose. You can also sense my emphasis or cry out to men in the world to care! Seriously, turn off your phones, get awake, stop being in charge and support your woman in this time of craze. Many fertility doctors and clinics require some kind of class before beginning the IVF process. Mine did. It is used to cut through all the confusion and give you a detailed picture of what you are getting yourself into. The class is given before a dime is taken, before a needle is pressed and before any inanimate objects are inserted into your "vajayjay" (as Oprah calls it).

I think it is a lot like entering the architectural, engineering or medical programs on our local college campus. The first few classes, so I hear, are created to weed out those who are not interested in putting in the long hours and really stretching their ability to absorb and retain large bits of information. I was a marketing and international business major, so I don't have a clue about weeding out but I picture this IVF "information" class to be much the same way. They scare the hell out of you with the truth and see who sticks around.

I left that stuffy, white, hospital conference room with sweaty palms and a brain pain. When Matt and I got to the car, we finally opened our mouths. He said "did you hear them say that, if it works, you take three months of daily shots?" I was so overloaded with other information that I totally missed that bit of wonderful news (sarcasm). We then had a one-hour car ride to discuss the entire process and those people involved.

Your spouse is a huge part of this fertility challenge. It may be your body that is having problems. It may be his. Goodness knows it may be both. But regardless of who is physically struggling, you are emotionally struggling TOGETHER.

This is your person you chose for better or worse and it is quite possible that this time of your life feels very much like "worse." It is necessary for you to communicate as much as your personality and marriage allows. The bumpy road becomes a lot smoother when you realize you are not traveling alone.

Matt and I met at a fraternity party at Oklahoma State University. I was a recently single junior out with my girlfriends two days before classes began and he was the president of his fraternity (hubba hubba). One glance at that guy gave me goose bumps. Being the lady I am, I was not about to make the first move. However, I positioned myself close to him all night and would be nearby should he want to chat. I would join in on conversations with mutual friends hoping for the possibility that he would direct the conversation onto me.

I wasn't a stalker or anything. I was just subtly making my presence known. Though not very smooth, these were all my best moves and he was not biting the hook. My girlfriends were jovially loving every minute of me being denied.

Finally, I noticed him talking to one of the girls I came with so I marched up to him with hands on hips and asked the question I knew would get a reaction. I asked him…

This isn't pretty. And if you are the kind of person who gets embarrassed for others, be prepared to be embarrassed for me.

… "Are you gay?"

I wish this was a joke. But alas, it is not. I was so foolishly enamored with myself that the only reason a man would not heap interest upon me like cool whip to an apple pie must be that he is gay. Looking back, the audacity of myself makes me cringe.

Fortunately, I got a response better than I had hoped for. I don't remember the quote but it went something like "no, and I'll prove it," followed by a kiss!

Now, I would rather our grandkids think we met at college on a lovely moonlit night while discussing something scholarly and that I was swept away merely by his intellect.

Truth be told. He was and still is a hottie! I was too forward. I was out late. I allowed him to kiss me too soon. Thank goodness for God's forgiveness and grace. (Can I get an Amen?)

We formed our relationship with dates and "hanging out," the way my generation does, until one day he came to me and announced, "I don't love you." I use the word "announced" because it was less of a discussion and more of a declaration. Now, I did not love him either. How could I? We were only a few months into dating. However, he was a senior in college and figured it was not worth wasting his time on a girl who he would not marry. Since he was not yet swept away in a fairy tale sort of way, he simply wanted to cut his losses.

This may sound rational, but not to the ears of the girl hearing it. I was devastated. How dare a man court me and then blow me off without really getting to know me?

He had been raised to look for a burst of fireworks or a puff of sparkling fairy dust when he met the woman that was made for him. He just assumed, like so many movies lead us to believe, that after meeting and creating your romantic story that your happily ever after moment is just that, an instantaneous, all comforting point of clarity in your declaration of life-long love. They left the part out about working to get there and working even harder to stay there.

My powers of negotiation kicked in. I'm not sure if I was negotiating our staying together because I already secretly loved him somewhere in my heart or because I was not about to let someone dump me.

Regardless, we decided to cut the fluff of dating and really get to know each other. We started not to talk about the movie we had just seen or what was on our dinner plate, but to talk about the fabric we were made of. We started to discuss God, our upbringing, our dreams, family, the stuff that really forms a person.

Turns out, we were made for one another and to this day, I joke with him about how he wanted to lose me and how I would not be lost. The first part of our story is definitely not fairy tale worthy but our romance became a whirlwind after that and we've had many more moments of greatness than points of frustration.

Our dates were so much fun. One night he took me for a motorcycle ride all over town. We drove through neighborhoods of homes in all sizes and talked about what we liked in the houses and didn't. Eventually, we came to a home under construction in a very nice neighborhood. We parked the bike and walked through it. It was becoming dusk, so we walked to the top floor and crawled out the window. We sat on the roof overlooking the city as the sun set.

Together, we decided there to exclusively date one another. Really, we had both already made that decision on our own, but had not verbalized that commitment to one another. This was a beautiful moment and one that puts me in a dreamy state every time I think about it.

Matt proposed to me exactly two years from the date we first met. (How better to memorialize the "are you gay" embarrassment?) He took me on that same motorcycle and into that same neighborhood that had since been gated and keypad coded. We entered with the code and drove up to that house. It had been completed for quite some time and a family lived there. We walked up to the wraparound front porch and came upon a beautiful setting. Two rocking chairs framed a table on which sat a vase of red roses, a bucket chilling Champagne and two burning candles. He got down on his knee and said something romantic and then opened the lighted box to display a ring.

I cannot recall the actual proposal. I was overwhelmed and sobbing. I had always known the right man would make the proposal perfectly. This captured all my heart.

It turns out the event was quite difficult for him to organize. He had to figure out who lived in the home and to contact them. Matt offered to buy them dinner if they would allow him the use of their porch for the evening. It turns out, that evening was their wedding anniversary and they planned to be out anyway. He prepared the rest of the scene on his own – flowers, candles, the whole shebang.

That was August and we were married the following April.

I believe when a person gets married, they should be required to do the following five things. Well, three are required readings. I was not a reader until a few years after college, so this reading list may seem daunting to those of you who are like I used to be. However, I would not call them "required" if I did not think they were valuable. Don't just read them, but do as they recommend. Here are those three books and the other two requirements for strengthening your marriage.

Say your vows in a church before God and your family and really mean them. Say "until death do us part" and genuinely make that commitment in spite of feelings and changes that are due your way. Life has its ups and downs, its awkward moments, its you-have-got-to-be-kidding-me situations and so do married relationships.

Marriage is not a commitment to be taken lightly. Far too many of my generation think they can undo a marriage like they undo the laces of a pair of brand new Nikes. Nothing could be further from the truth. Make this true commitment and then, if you have to, fight like a wild turkey to keep it.

When bumps come your way, find a fix, talk to a professional, have date night, buy *The Love Dare* book, try hard to remember why you fell in love. Do all you can to keep those vows! Without this foundation, you should not be attempting to have a child.

For good communication advice and tips read the book *Men are from Mars, Women are from Venus*. Both husband and wife should be required to read this book. This book is a joyful reminder that we are made differently from one another but formed this way so that we fit together. It not only gives you an understanding of yourself and your partner, but it allows you a new vocabulary for communication. I can come home to my husband when he is in the most funky mood and all he has to say is "honey, I need to go into my cave."

To the unfamiliar ear, this may sound a little vampire/batman–ish when, in fact, I understand him to be saying "I need some time alone to stew in the juices of what is going on in my work world. Then I can come back to you happy and normal. And this has absolutely nothing to do with you or us." That's just one example of how it just helps you understand each other better which alleviates a multitude of other issues. This book should be required reading. I personally own four copies of this book, none of which are currently in my home library because I regularly lend them to friends.

Read *The Five Love Languages*. Wow, this book should be a classic. I'm not sure how you get on the classics list, but it should be somewhere next to *Tom Sawyer* and *To Kill A Mockingbird*. It should be among the books that you are given at birth in leather bound covers.

It describes how people love in one of five different ways. The reader is encouraged to figure out which one she is and share that with her spouse and friends. The deal is, you may feel like you're expressing love to someone by telling them over and over, but if "Words of Affirmation" is not their "love language," they may completely miss your expression.

If you know one another's love language and attempt to communicate to each other accordingly, your spouse will be affirmed and reciprocate love back. Thus, you maintain or grow a healthy relationship and learn to communicate better. It is brilliant.

My love language is "Acts of Service" and Matt's is "Words of Affirmation" mixed with "Physical Touch." To show love, I tell him how handsome he is and he does the dishes for me. Two of my best friends are "Quality Time," and my sister-in-law is "Gifts." Now that I know how they experience love, I can share with them how much I love them by "speaking" their love language. Genius – right? This book has one of those "duh" factors, which is an excellent sign of a great advice book. Read it!

Yet another book that should be instantly read upon the words "yes, I will marry you, thanks for the big fat diamond" is the book *Rocking the Roles*. If you, like me, cringe at the Biblical word "submit," this is the book for you. It will change your perspective as well as give you a new point of view probably never before considered.

If you don't know what role you should or want to play as wife and mother, you better get that figured out. Hubbies need to know their job and we need to know ours. Businesses, small and large, give their employees titles so that you know what they are supposed to be doing within the walls of the office. We are given the title "husband" and "wife" so that we know our roles also. This does not mean that the wife has to do all the cooking and the husband gets to sit on the couch drinking his Budweiser. It means that, together, you must figure out who will do what and when that will take place so that your home and family can function in a smooth manner. No marriage will look or function like any other. You have to figure out for both of you who does what and what works for you as a couple.

*Journal Entry*
> *We women have a special role in this world. We have a capacity to love and feel that is greater than the mighty oceans. We have a calling to love each other with all of our hearts and souls. We have the ability to cry when something is sad and laugh when something is funny. We are able to be strong and sensitive, mysterious and real. We are the ones who build the cities after the construction is finished. We live with our hearts exposed because we do not know another way.*

This makes us beautifully different than our men and sadly vulnerable. I believe my husband loves me because I need him and he needs me. Give a man a jar to open and they will feel like a king for the afternoon. Become completely independent and they'll sense you wondering "why have him around?" I have learned that submitting to my husband (in terms of the way I express respect) empowers us both.

Work every day at being in love. As we have all heard, love is not a feeling – it is an action. This is so very true. In the midst of the I word, you cannot loose sight of what you are doing. You are trying to take a tiny part of him and mix it with a tiny part of you and give to the world a beautiful gift. You feel so passionately about how wonderful a man you have found that you plan to combine the very best part of him with the very best part of you and make a blessed creation that you will love in a way no one will ever be able to describe.

Working at your love starts out much like the first day at a new job. You are awkward, running late, not sure what you are supposed to do and you can't find the coffee pot. Sooner or later, you figure out why you submitted your application and accepted the offer. You eventually become good at what you do. The same is true for loving someone... or loving them again. Put notes on their steamy bathroom mirror. Send a love text. Shoot a sappy one liner email. Make dessert. Grab his hand while you walk to the car. Buy his favorite gum instead of your favorite gum. Sit on the back porch and listen to his story about the egg head guy in the accounting department. You get the point.

That's it. These five steps don't guarantee a perfect marriage but they do encourage a strong one and get you started in the habit of working on your marriage. Another book that's been highly recommended to me is called *For Women Only*, by Shaunti Feldhahn, which highlights great insights into our men. There is so much out there to help you learn and grow and challenge yourself to be a strong wife and have a healthy marriage. You deserve to make that investment in yourself and in the life of your future child's parents! You've heard people say that you have to be strong on your own before you can be ok in marriage. Likewise that you need to be ok in your marriage before you can get through this fight for a family.

Another note about our personal story: We both wanted children but wanted to spend time as newlyweds for a while first. So, I remained on the birth control pill, which I had taken since I was 15. As a teen, I had irregular periods that were quite painful, so the doctor regulated me this way. Then I needed it for contraception reasons of course.

Time passed in our marriage and the conversation of children came up now and again. I decided that I wanted him to make the decision of when we should stop birth control. I wasn't totally ready to be a mom (in fact, it scared the curse words out of me), but I knew when it happened it would all work out. So, we came up with a plan; our own code for jump starting that part of our lives.

A business associate and friend of Matt's lives in South Africa and had recently come to Oklahoma for a visit. He brought a bottle of wine made in his country. We wanted "the decision" to be memorable, so we made that bottle of wine our code. He would open it and pour us both a glass when he was ready to officially start trying to have a child.

I received that glass of wine in late December 2003. Strangely enough, that was the most terrible glass of wine we have ever put to our lips. In fact, after our first glass, we poured the entire bottle down the drain of our kitchen sink. We then embraced, kissed, kitchen danced and went to the bedroom to start what became a very long, discouraging but eventually victorious journey.

I really do think I have an especially blessed marriage. This is what makes writing this section tricky for me. I don't need a ton of advice on how to talk to my husband and he does not need words to teach him how to respond to my needs. I also know that my situation is unique. Even with dream boat Matt, there are stressful marriage days that evolve from my uproar of emotion or days when he just doesn't say the right thing, try as he may.

There is a Web site called www.BabyHopes.com and they have a free email newsletter called "Trying to Conceive." It is a simple little newsletter but there are some good snipits of info in there. In a recent newsletter there was an article about dealing with fertility as a couple.

Here is what it said:

*Facing Marital Problems While Going Through Fertility
Treatments*

*Having treatments for fertility can be an arduous experience.
Going through fertility treatments can also be an emotional roller
coaster, which can affect every area of a couples' lives. Many
couples even find themselves facing marital problems while going
through fertility treatments. Fortunately, there are some things that
couples can do to avoid these problems, as well as things that can
help them face marital problems should they arise.*

*The key to any successful relationship, personal or professional,
is communication. Couples who are going through fertility
treatments need to make sure that they are communicating how
they feel to their partner and that they are actively listening to
their partner's feelings. It is true that fertility treatments, especially
when they are not successful, can be extremely disappointing and
lead to emotions of hopelessness, anxiety and even anger. It is
likely that your spouse is feeling these things as well. By making
your spouse a real partner in facing these emotions, you can help
to avoid having marital problems.*

*Another big cause of marital problems while going through fertility
treatments is stress. Anxiety makes us all at least a little bit crabby
from time to time. While going through fertility treatments, it is
important that couples practice stress management techniques.
They should be sure to exercise regularly, to eat a diet low in
caffeine and low in fats and to make sure that they are getting
enough sleep. Many marital problems, whether when going
through fertility treatments or not, can be attributed to a plain old
lack of sleep.*

*Therapy may also help couples face marital problems when they
are going through fertility treatments. A marital therapist can often
help couples who otherwise have trouble communicating with one
another to explore their feelings and to find common ground. Far
from being a last resort, couples should view marital counseling as*

*a part of the big picture of their fertility treatments.*

*While there is not a magic potion that can help you face marital problems while going through fertility treatments, practicing these principles may help you to get through the rough times together, as a couple.*

I thought it was general information, but nonetheless, good.

Bottom line, having a child is not going to improve your marriage. It is not going to help you fit in with all your friends who are also having children. It is not going to make you something you are not already. In fact, it will test your marital strength. It will force you to squeeze a bit more time into Thursday so that you can lay eyes on your best friend. It will make you accidentally expose your breast to an entire restaurant so that your child can eat. It will make you miss those nights on the couch when you wished you had something better to do.

Parenting is not done well by a couple that constantly argues. Don't get me wrong, I know plenty of people who make it work. I also know plenty of people who are single parents or who might as well be single parents for all the help that DON'T get from their supposed mate. But that is what they do - make it work.

There is a huge difference between the stability of parenting when it is single sided versus two fully involved people working together for the best interest of a child without arguing regularly or even throwing extended absences into the norm of their lives. This makes a difference in the well being for the child, but also for the parent(s).

I can't imagine how difficult it is to be on your own with a child or two or three constantly in tow. I applaud my mother who did just that. A girl needs her breather and having a healthy marriage relationship gives mommy that time. It also gives the child invaluable daddy time. Some friends have a strong enough marriage. They may not call their husband "dream boat" as I refer to Matt. One friend, for example, remembers the numb feeling that struck her with an immeasurable weight as she began to question her marriage during infertility treatments.

She recalls that, as they waited in the ultrasound room, suspecting bad news, her sweet husband leaned close to her face and said, "It's ok, no matter what. I'm ok if it's just you and me all of our lives. I love you." His heart just wanted to comfort hers and she was unable to reciprocate the level of love. That heartbreaking moment of motherhood fears left her shaken to the core. She wondered if she loved her husband enough or even at all. My friend wondered if bringing a baby into the world may be a mistake.

Wisely, she worked through this and recognized the hormone-induced, stress-riddled state she was in may not have allowed her to instantaneously express love for and contentment with her husband. She explored her heart and intentionally focused on his positive traits so she could heal at the deepest level. They are all (three now) doing excellently, although she would still roll her eyes if you tried to call her marriage "strong."

No marriage is perfect and you might not even think yours is great. However, you made the commitment and your marriage deserves you investing some effort and energy. If not, pains of fertility complications and other life stresses are infinitely multiplied.

My point clearly is to have a good marriage BEFORE expanding the population.

In a recent phone conversation while I was home in Oklahoma and my friend (who is struggling for a family) was traveling in Florida, I asked if she had been enjoying all this travel for work. She said that it has been fun, but that was not her real reason for packing on the hours away. She admitted that she needs to travel. If she stays home she sulks and spends far more time thinking about her "problem." Running away from the situation is rarely a good way to handle something.

She also said that her husband asked her to stop traveling so much. He missed her and wanted her home with him. She unveiled the truth and told him why she wanted to travel. He understood but he wanted to deal with it together. Now that is a good man! He wants to be with his wife. I pray that she feels rewarded for the man she has.

It is very much like us women to become reclusive when things aren't going our way, but we must not dismiss our husbands. Instead, it is into his arms that we should be running. You have created a partnership, so allow him to be as involved as he can be. If he is a computer junkie like my husband, then turn him loose on research for causes, treatments and new information. If he is a Godly man, pray with him and let him lead you through scriptural promises. If he is hands on with no qualms about giving shots, then let him help you with that.

If he is none of these and doesn't want to talk about it, invest in staying alongside him until you find your ways to communicate and partner on this. He may love you and hurt for you but he may not want to listen to you whine, put shots in your butt, pray for you, read with you or research babies. The women in that IVF informational class, whose husbands I was slamming, deserve babies as much as a woman with a seemingly more devoted man. We all deserve kids. There are moments where we'll all feel like we don't. We will all have moments where we feel like our marriage isn't ready.

Regardless of your current marital state, my challenge to you is simple. Don't make this experience something that isolates you from your husband. Make it one that brings you two together in new ways. More than likely, he is just as eager to become a father as you are to become a mother (only he is a dude and they don't really talk like that).

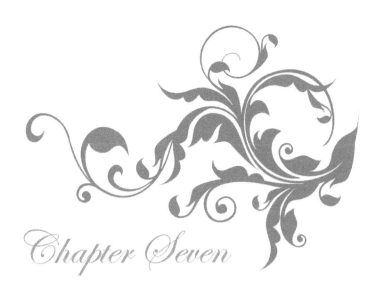

# MORALITY AND MEDICINE

*A*s noted in the advice section of "Control Your Own Care," you may come to a crossroads in your treatment plan when you will ask yourself "how far down the road of fertility enhancements am I willing to go?"

*Journal Entry*
> *I am not sure if the first day I began this journal I expressed how difficult the decision to try IVF was for me. It is one of the most difficult decisions I have made to date. I do not want to interfere with God's master plan and I want to interpret the "signs" correctly. I assume stepping on God's toes is a dangerous path. Well, now we are at a similar crossroads and my emotions are yet again tied into knots along with my moral and ethical questions - just like a roll of Christmas lights that may never be untangled.*

When I was a child of about eight living in a small town in Alaska with my mom and stepfather, I had a conversation over a cup of hot chocolate next to a fire that would mold my spiritual outlook until I was 20. I'm not sure if I was an inquisitive child or just a talkative one, but the question of "why" was frequent spewing from my lips. I do not know the exact wording of my question, but I asked my stepfather about God. His response was that "God is the answer to questions that people do not know the answer to."

Philosophically speaking, he may not have been wrong. Why is the sky blue? God made it that way. Why does grandma have to die? God has a plan that is unknown to us.

But to a malleable elementary school child, this was an opportunity to share the gospel - if only it was believed in my childhood home. Instead, I took this response to mean that God was not real. God was what big people said instead of "I don't know." It made me debate Christian believers in my youth. I have a gift for persuasion in a heated argument or debate and this came in quite handy to prove to the undereducated believer that she did not know what she was talking about.

When I met my husband in 1998, he was a Christian and I, of course, was not. After dating a few weeks, he asked to take me to church. I was terrified! I had two vivid memories of church. The first was when my precious doll was "stolen." Looking back, I probably left the doll in a pew and took off in my patent leather shoes after a relative.

The second was when I stayed with a friend on a Saturday night and thus was required to attend church with the family the following morning. Their church had burned to the ground about six months prior so the congregation was holding service outside in a beautiful wooded area in the lot next to the church's reconstruction.

I remember little of the service until I noticed that each row of wooden pews was slowly emptying. The once seated figures were raising and walking to the front of the church, doing something and then returning to their seats. I was not about to join this march. However, the mother of my girlfriend gingerly pushed me along.

Upon arriving at the front of the makeshift church, where every single eye seemed to fall upon my uncomfortable and terrified preteen frame,

I was offered a cup and a biscuit. I had watched TV accounts of this before and had carefully studied the person in front of me, so I knew what I was supposed to do. However, I had never before, and have never since, experienced what happened next.

The people finished their juice, ate their tasteless biscuit, took a few more steps and stood in front of a cross. The man holding the cross smiled with sweet eyes as the congregation, one at a time, kissed the center of the cross. I was more uncomfortable than I can ever remember being but I did not want to make a scene, so I took my steps, closed my eyes and kissed.

I did not pause, however, between the stepping and the kissing and sort of bumped my nose into the cross. No one, except the cross holder, my friend in front and her mother behind saw me, though it felt as though it was broadcast live at the Super Bowl. To add insult to mild injury, my friend said to me "you are not supposed to run your face into it." As any young preteen girl would be, I was mortified. This event reminded me, one more time, that I was not suited for church.

So, there I was, scheduled for that church date with Matt and I was understandably scared. What does a 20-year-old girl do when she is scared? She has her college roommate come along, of course. That is exactly what I did. We were going to a Presbyterian church. She was a Catholic and I was... trembling.

We went and nothing embarrassing, humiliating or life altering happened. Praise God! I spent most of the church time fighting the faith. Rolling my eyes when we would talk about salvation and making a slight disgusted look when we would sing about the blood of Jesus. This was not my saving moment but for a guy to get me in those doors was a big step.

As time went on, Matt asked me questions like "what do you believe about angels," and "what do you think happens when you die." These open ended conversations shared without judgment allowed him to walk me slowly to Christ.

We went "church shopping" for months as a seriously dating couple. I was not yet a Christian but was also not opposed to the possibility at this point. Eventually, we found a place we still call home and I made an appointment to meet with the pastor. I planned for weeks by making a list of all my questions, all my debate points, all my apprehensions. I was frank and so was he (actually he was JB and I was Kristine, but you get my point). I loved it.

I am not sure if the following event happened while leaving that meeting or several weeks later, but I know it was somewhere close by. I was about to graduate from college and had a big fat decision to make: do I pack my bags and take on the world solo or do I try to find employment in the town where Matt is working? I knew I loved him, but I was not sure if we were going to get married, have a house, make babies and live happily ever after – though I hoped so.

I remember driving north on Duck Street between Hall of Fame and McElroy, listening to the radio on a cloudy, but not stormy, day. I was thinking hard about this decision and the implications that it could have on my life. Just then, I see the red and blue lights of a patrol car flashing in my rear view mirror. My mind had been on autopilot and my foot had been on the gas.

I pulled over, handed the officer my information and waited with my hands on the wheel. As I lay my head back on the rest I prayed "God what do I do with my life?" And that is when it happened.

I was listening to country music and my radio cut out slightly. Then a portion of the Mark Wills song came on and said "All things in time, time will reveal." The music cut out for just a fraction of a second again before returning to fluidly streaming in the rest of the song. My breath was gone and I knew that God and I were beginning to make connection in the depths of my heart. I was consumed with an attraction to His truth and excitedly anticipating the next steps He was guiding me to take.

In that moment it seemed that He had found a way to slow me down, literally pull me over and capture my full attention. He had answered my question about Matt and so many of my questions about Christ. The clarity I felt for the Lord after that was spectacular. I finally understood Jesus' parables as I studied. I became a Christian.

I was as ignorant, green and naive as a person could be. I was also terrified because of all the Christian-bashing I had done the 21 years before. With time, I learned. I continue to learn. I read the story of Paul who, as he was on his way to KILL Christians, was saved through faith. I knew that if Paul and all the wretched things he did could be forgiven, then I could be forgiven too. My life changed. My outlook changed. My future changed. I stayed in the college town where Matt worked, attended church with him and continued to nurture the newfound love for my Savior.

Those of you who are Christians may realize why I am giving you my story of believing and where I am going with this. Regardless of your faith, there is a moral dilemma involved with family planning. You question yourself as to where the line is drawn. Are you supposed to make a plan or do you just have sex and see what God wants for you? And if you decide to use medical science, just how far with it do you go? Did God create me to be born in this era of medical advancements so that I could proceed down this journey? What is "right," here and how is that defined for me spiritually?

When I was going through my "challenge," Nicole was one of my confidants and now I am one of hers. It is a true joy to me to be able to relate to her trials. I pray with and for Nicole. I listen when she needs me to just hear her and I talk when I have something valuable to add. (Actually, I just talk whenever I want – I just hope that something valuable is coming out.)

Recently we sat curled up on the gray couch in my maroon living room and discussed this exact issue. She is at the point in her "fight" where she needs to decide what steps to take next. She has done the Clomid thing and now has to decide if she should move to something more aggressive. Her personal battle is deeply rooted in her faith. She has spoken to God numerous times (every hour) asking for guidance. As of this day, she has not yet received those signs.

It is obvious, being the outsider, that she is growing very close to God through this experience. She is constantly seeking His will and trusting that her actions are not contrary to His will. Before I became a believer, I remember thinking "if I'm wrong and there is a God, I don't want to piss him off." Both views require legitimate and thorough introspection as to what you should do.

In our discussion, Nicole reminded me yet again of the very raw emotion of abandonment. You want to ask God "why are you doing this to me?" or "what have I done wrong?" You want to make deals and bets with God like "If you give me a child, I will never watch soap operas again," or "God, if I hear my favorite song on the radio in the next hour, then I will know you are telling me to take the next step."

As a note from personal experience, this doesn't work. Give it a whirl if you want to. You probably should be doing something better with your time than watching soaps anyway, but don't think that you will magically become pregnant because of the sacrifice or God bargaining.

This may be the first time in your life that you have questioned God and your faith. It is very scary, but understandable.

Let me tell you what you need to hear most of all. God is not abandoning you. You did nothing wrong. This is not your fault. You are not alone.

In the first chapter of her book, *Eight Choices That Will Change a Woman's Life*, Jill Briscoe says, "If we ask angrily, 'What is this trouble doing in my life?' we have not realized that the trouble we are suffering is acceptable to the Lord and therefore should be acceptable to us." She follows this later in the chapter with this wonderful analogy.

"Pain can make us ready for God. When do we most urgently seek the

Almighty? I suspect it is when trouble intrudes itself into our peaceful lives and we need his guidance and wisdom.

A traveler reading a book on a train noticed a friendly little girl playing around the seats, talking to the other passengers and showing them her toys. The traveler put down his book and exchanged a few words with her, wondering whom she belonged to. She seemed perfectly at ease with everyone, so it was hard to tell. Suddenly the train entered a long, dark tunnel and the lights flickered. The traveler smiled when the little girl darted toward a man sitting at the end of the carriage and flung herself into his arms. There was no doubt to whom she belonged.

The world constantly watches those of us who love Jesus. Perhaps they wonder to whom we belong. While everything is going well, it may be hard to tell. But let us enter a long, dark tunnel and there will be absolutely no doubt. They will watch us dive into the arms of God and then they will know! Just as surely as suffering gets us ready for Him, it also alerts a watching world to a source of help they know nothing about. There are many travelers on the train of life who need to see that happen."

You would not think that the Bible could relate to the question of how far to go with medically induced pregnancy. Truly, it does not tell you what to do in exact wording but it does remind you that you are not alone in this matter or any matter of your heart. Your fight for a family is not a new battle. You have sisters engaged in this battle all the way back to the first people who roamed the earth. Find comfort in that. God gave them a reason for the battle that isn't immediately clear in the scriptures. The same is true with you.

As I said, I had a personal, Christian struggle in my decision making. Like many girls of my generation, I sought out the opinions of my girlfriends. A friend (now my sister-in-law) was living in Florida at the height of my plight. Therefore, she was removed from the daily ups and downs of the decision making process. One afternoon, I shot her a long and detailed email about the difficulties of decision making. Her response is a story that I have taken with me every day:

A man is sitting in his house and the floodwater is rising fast. A rescue worker arrives in a row boat and invites the man to come to safety. "No thanks," the man says "God will save me." The rescue worker leaves and the waters continue to rise. The man moves to the roof where he is met by a helicopter. "Climb in, we will take you to safety," the helicopter pilot says. "No thanks," the man says again "God will save me." The man drowns.

Upon arriving in heaven the man is confused. "I had faith that you would save me God, why am I here?" the man asks. And God responds, "I sent you a boat and a helicopter."

Only you can decide when and if you want to be "rescued" from your current predicament. Only your personal prayer time, Bible study and long talks with your husband will guide you to what's right for your family.

When going through our situation, we learned about the thousands of procedures and medications available for procreation assistance. I used to think that the medical profession was very dry. A patient has this problem, the doctor prescribes this medication. The opposite is true. The medical profession truly is an art.

I once joked with our doctor about how left handed folks are supposed to be in more creative lines of work. He's left handed so I jokingly inquired about his profession. He told me seriously that there are few professions that require more daily creativity than medicine. Depending on your age, condition, situation and eagerness, a different formula can be manipulated.

For fun, let's start from the beginning and discuss just a smidgen about each of the "leaps" or "phases" you might consider in your battle with the I word.

As we go though these procedures, remember that I will skip several, joke about all and try my hardest not to advise you in any way about when you should take the next leap. I am here to share one story – my story - that gives you something to relate to, something to be inspired by and something to learn from as you walk through this maze.

First, there is sex. Good old fashioned getting it on until the break of dawn, no thought to how ripe his semen is and when you may be ovulating. It is just a matter of attraction. You think he is hot. He thinks you are sexy. He took out the garbage this morning. You finished your errands. The stars are in alignment and you had a glass of wine, so it's boom boom time.

This is the ideal means to the requested end of course, but if you are reading this book, it is probably not your means. You don't have to worry about the moral aspect of sperm meeting egg unless you are unmarried or un-in-love, both of which are other books subjects for other times by other authors.

Second, and maybe I should not be numbering these because as we get further down the line the order becomes grayed, is also doctor-less sex but with heightened information. There are countless Web sites and books available that detail temperature spikes, mucus checking and other ovulation-related goo.

A few of my good friends used a book about taking charge of your fertility. One used the book to help her understand her fertility, so she knew when to make the whoopee to make a baby and the other used it as a birth control method. Strangely enough, the one wanting to get pregnant still is not and the one trying to control pregnancy got "knocked up". Don't worry, she is happily married and all is well.

I don't believe either situation is a result of the book (it is probably an excellent read but apparently it's not a sure fix). In fact, I have yet another friend who used the same information to try to ensure that she would have a girl because she already had two sons. That worked. This gets into an entirely separate discussion about gender preferences, of which I am not at all interested.

Nonetheless, understanding your body is one way to rev up the possibility of getting pregnant and I don't think there are any moral battles that are waged over understanding your ovulation in order to assist the process.

My guess is that this is when the seeds of frustration begins to grow roots. You start saying to yourself "oh crap, am I going to be one of those?" This might be the time you go in to your regular ObGyn and ask for the litany of tests and evaluations that may determine why you are not like every drunken cheerleader getting pregnant in the midst of wild, crazy fun.

Personally, when the tests came back with no obvious problems, the next step offered to us was the use of a medication called Clomid. Its job description is to increase the number and size of the eggs you release each month in order to help your procreation chances. Instead of those zillion sperms battling the canal towards one single teensy egg, with Clomid the sperm have a larger reward once they get to the promised land. Here is where the slope of morality can begin to slide. You are now using science to increase your chances.

For me, this was a no-brainer. We use medication to stop cold symptoms, provide us our vitamins and remove headaches. What is the big deal with one to give me super ovulation? For many folks, this is when you need to start having the discussion with your spouse. You want the Clomid to work, but what if it doesn't? How many months will you try it? It is important to begin discussing just how far you are willing to go and at what pace.

I'm sure there are 84,000 steps between this and the next, but again, I am not a medical professional and won't pretend to be. I'm just a girl with a personal situation. However, when talking with my regular ObGyn, I learned that it is at this point that a woman should see a Reproductive Endocrinology and Infertility specialist, a medical doctor known in the industry as an REI. These are your specialists, the ones with the education, experience and equipment for making you a parent. I highly recommend that if you are seeking treatment for infertility that you at least entertain the idea of seeing someone whose training and daily grind includes getting women pregnant, not checking the paps and delivering the babies.

I know you are immediately concerned about switching doctors and potentially offending your regular doc. My ObGyn assures me that this is a silly concern. If a doctor discourages your seeing someone else so that he or she can keep you in that practice, then I would be highly skeptical.

If you love your ObGyn and don't want to leave him, then go get yourself pregnant and then have him handle your pregnancy and birth. Those are the fun visits anyway.

Next on our list of possible procedures is IUI (Intrauterine Insemination), or in layman's terms taking the sperm, cleaning out all the gunk and putting it into the uterus with a turkey baster of sorts. I believe there is more to it than this, but the general idea is there. The good part about IUI is that, in the grand scheme of things, it is not too cost prohibitive and quite effective for many folks.

Assuming you have exhausted all "easy" and economically manageable procedures, next is In Vitro Fertilization or IVF. This basically involves shooting your bottom with a million needles in order to grow your eggs and to create a hospitable environment for baby growth. Then, the doctor takes the sperm and cleans it up as discussed above with IUI. They remove the eggs from your body and mix it with your husband's sperm and then watch it grow in a dish for three to five days before putting a few back in your uterus to see what "takes" and becomes a growing baby fetus. This is followed by lots and lots and lots of prayer.

Now, if your sperm aren't as wiggly as they need to be to do the Petri dish trick, then there is a process called "ICSI", which is pronounced "ick-see" and I have no idea what it stands for. It has something to do with figuring out which of the billions of teensy sperm are super sperm, pulling them out of the bunch and placing them directly into the egg. This way, the sperm do not have to do any work to get to the egg. It is just plucked from its friends and stuck in there. This alleviates the concern that the sperm won't find their way to their "home."

If your eggs are fine and your sperm are the problem for what ever reason, you could also consider a sperm donor. Most people have heard of this because it is the butt of every college boy's joke.

Guy 1: "I don't have money for beer, so I will just go to the bank and make a deposit."

Guy 2: "Which bank?"

Guy 1: "The sperm bank." Ha Ha Ha

Girl in the car with these two guys: audible sigh and rolling eyes.

But, if your hubby had testicular cancer and his sperm won't swim or you're missing a testicle like the guy in the movie *While You Were Sleeping* or your partner has some hereditary disease he does not want to pass along or any of the billions of other less scary reasons for unusable sperm, then sperm donation is something you may need to know about.

On the same playing field as sperm donation, which many of us may be unaware of, is egg donation. This is where some woman, as an egg donor, basically experiences the first part of IVF by getting all the shots and taking all the medication to grow her eggs. Then, instead of fertilizing them and putting them back into her own uterus, they are fertilized with your husband's sperm and put into your body.

If you are learning about IVF for the first time, you will probably not realize what I have just said. If you are an IVF information veteran, then you get this. This egg donor woman is willing to put her body through countless shots in the tummy and hiney, take a menagerie of hormone inducing pills and undergo outpatient surgery that requires anesthesia –

all for a woman she has never met and never will meet! Men can just think happy thoughts into their specimen cup. Their donation is easy breezy compared to the serious business of the egg donation.

It is interesting to think about the women who make themselves available for this kind of thing. Regardless of why they choose to undergo all the physical stress, they are amazing women. Maybe some do it for the money but for all the work, pain and potential complications, there really is not a lot of money in it. I asked Karen, the wonder nurse, about this and she described a VERY in depth screening process including phases of medical as well as emotional tests. These women are devoted to helping other women where they cannot help themselves. Whatever their reason for donating, they are helping other women feel like women and ultimately become mothers.

Can you imagine the doctor telling you that your eggs are broken? If you have experienced this, I am so very sorry! I picture feeling gypped for enduring all the periods of my life for a big fat nothing. Then there are a few selfless women who know how important this gift could be to a woman who otherwise would have broken eggs and broken motherhood dreams.

I suppose the same is true for men. Hearing that your sperm won't wiggle has to feel emasculating even though no one in the world would see it that way except for the man hearing it. Again, I am so sorry if this is a part of your uphill fertility climb. If either of you is in the situation and feeling robbed, that is because you are! It is my opinion that God has reasons and plans for this, but feeling cheated seems like a perfectly acceptable emotion for a short time.

I don't think the obvious morality battle over donations and the receipt of those donations needs to be highlighted. Like so many of these decisions, this is a very personal issue and one that no one can judge until put in that situation.

My husband and I had a conversation about egg and sperm donation over dinner one night and he commented that the child may have been created in an unconventional way, but the life of every child is given not by the blood of its parents, but by their heart. How very true!

After learning about these donations, I spoke to our nurse about the other interesting options we, the fertility-challenged couples of this day and age, have available to us. Here are a few more on the sliding scale of medical assistance.

If the female body is unable to carry a child for any number of reasons, but her eggs are strong and his sperm are wiggling, then there is also what I will call "uterus donation" to keep standardized with the sperm and egg donation terms used above. It is really called a surrogate mother. (My husband hates it when I invent new words or phrases, but you get it, right?)

I have a girlfriend who is considering being the uterus donor for a friend of hers from college. My friend has had three wonderful children and has had her tubes tied. She is finished creating her family. Her college friend, however, has some kind of heart condition and surgical complication from childhood that eliminates her ability to carry a child.

When discussing this with my friend, she said she feels "made for it". Her pregnancies were very healthy and easy. She actually enjoyed being pregnant. She is an amazing mother, but she isn't the type that really connects with her babies until they breathe their first breaths. She monitors her health of course, but she's not one to really bond with the idea of the baby until she meets the little wonder. She never personally understood why she was this way until her college friend mentioned her potential need for surrogate motherhood. Maybe she doesn't connect during pregnancy because she'd be emotionally stable to give a newborn to another mother that way. God prepares us all for different roles in each other's lives. His plan is ever amazing and baffling to me.

From the college friend's perspective, she will know that the child would be grown in a wonderful environment by someone who does not smoke, drink, do drugs, or work with weird radiation. She knows that the baby would be prayed over constantly. She would also feel invited and welcomed at every check up without awkward fears.

This is such a personal decision and one that both parties will make independent of one another. How wonderful that there are women out there who believe so greatly in the power of motherhood that they are willing to give up nine plus months of their life to help a sister in need? I celebrate this selfless act!

There is also the situation where his sperm and your eggs are both broken, but your body is able to carry a child. In that case, there is embryo donation. This can happen when IVF "patients" have completed the fertility process and created their family to fit their desires. However, the IVF process is not an exact science and a couple may have remaining embryos that are kept frozen. These couples can decide to put the embryos up for "adoption."

As I understand it, the process works very much like sperm and egg donation where a couple reviews the paperwork of the couples that have embryos to spare. The wanna-be parents pick the genetics that coordinate with the hair and eye color, interests, height and talents – if available and if the recipient wishes. Then the female body is prepared much the same way as IVF or egg donation. The embryos are then thawed and placed in your body for growth. The embryo donors may be told that their embryos have gone to a wonderful couple, but no further information is given – ever.

Adoption of any sort is an amazing option to consider. Whether you choose to consider domestic adoption or international adoption, welcoming a child into your heart and your home is a priceless honor; an opportunity unlike any other. I hear story after story about wonderful adoption experiences, as well as statistically proven risks for adoption. Consider it, research it and study it. May God bless the birth mothers who carry their children to term and give those babies a chance! And may God bless the families that take that chance and turn it into loving life.

I am sure that I have missed about ninety other situations, operations and procedures, but that is not the point I am trying to drive home. The point I want to make is that this is an individual decision based on your individual circumstance, belief, financial ability and comfort level. You MUST talk about all the options as they arrive on your plate.

The emotion involved with any of these steps is difficult. If you are at the stage of only six months ago flushing your birth control pills down the toilet and are reading this upon your first action of putting pillows under your bottom after having sex, then you know the anticipation. For those of you who have slid down the scale of medical decision-making like me, you painfully understand the emotion and trials that are involved.

Again, I am so sorry that you have to go through this. What crap it is that we even have to make these kinds of decisions. Before I was "fertility-challenged" I had a hard time deciding where I wanted to eat. Now these magnanimous decisions become ours to make.

These decisions are hard to make, but make them and then stick by them. Like Nike says "just do it," what ever "it" may be for you.

Remember this is a very personal decision. Don't let anyone make these decisions for you. Don't do anything you would regret later and don't skip anything you wish you would have tried. This is YOUR experience (with all its yucky-ness). Be in charge. And good luck.

# FEEL IT UP

*M*att and I, along with his family, purchased some ranch land west of town. I did not know a single thing about owning a ranch but, like it or not, I was about to learn. We purchased a few head of Brahman cattle from this sale and a few Angus cattle from that sale. It was our goal to form a new genetic line of Brangus animals. Therefore, we were taking the best genetics from the Brahman world of breeding and mixing it with the best genetics of the Angus world to produce (several years from now) our own beautiful Brangus creatures (which are 3/8 Brahman and 5/8 Angus – you will not be required to do any more math today).

You don't have to slap on your cowboy boots and wranglers to read this chapter, stick with me.

In order to form these genetics, there are a ton of high tech fertility manipulation techniques that take place. We gave shots to our heifers (girl cows that haven't had babies – like one of us) to super ovulate. We bought semen from top bulls and artificially inseminated the heifers. The animals are then "preg checked" a few months later to see if it worked. Sound familiar to any of you who've already started treatments?

Our ranch has not yet gone down this route, but many high end ranch operations find a cow (girl cow that has had babies – a mom) with fantastic genetics regarding low birth weight, fast growth, a good rump roast, whatever and have her injected with fertility drugs in order to produce tons of eggs. They will remove the eggs from the animal, pick a high quality sperm donor bull and, with the magic of a Petri dish, make embryos. Then they will take these embryos and implant them into mediocre cows (or heifers) for gestation and birth. She's a surrogate mother of sorts. This way the cow with "good genetics" can essentially have several babies in one year.

Had you any idea that the cattle industry was so advanced in fertility? Yeah, me neither. But, because of our personal circumstances, I needed little explanation as to what was going on.

When an animal does not get pregnant through these methods, she is sent out into a pasture with a "clean up bull." This animal has the best job in the world. His life goal is to sex up all these non-pregnant heifers and cows until they are pregnant. They also get to eat a lot. Pretty much, the clean up bull has the job every American male wishes he had, with the exception that the clean up bull does not get to watch football or eat Doritos. Though, I am sure that given the chance, a clean up bull would do both. We currently have two lucky bulls on our land. The Brahman bull is named Booger (or at least that is what I call him). The Angus bull is creatively called "Angus bull."

I started noticing, several months after Artificially Inseminating (AI-ing) our heifers that one was put into "the garden." This is a small fenced section of our property near the house that will eventually become a produce garden.

At that time, we did not have so many animals on the ranch that they ran together in my mind. So, I knew that this specific animal didn't get pregnant from the AI and had been with either Booger or the Angus Bull for the last couple of months.

"What is the deal with number 587," I asked my husband.

"She's infertile," he responded.

"So why is she in the garden?"

"We are going to fatten her up and butcher her," was his easy response. Then he grinned while adding, "We have named her 'ribeye.'"

My heart started pounding and my mind started racing. My family is going to kill an animal because she is infertile. I was heartbroken and my mouth immediately went to the irrational comment of "are you sure you don't want to put me down while you are at it!?"

I know now and knew then that my reaction was ridiculous. Cattle are produced in this country for beef and I love a good ribeye, lightly seasoned, cooked medium rare over an open flame. But this was personal.

I identified with this animal. It had tried regular sex and fertility drugs and neither of them had produced conception. Number 587 was on the same path I was on and she was going to be eaten for dinner.

She is still in the garden and is fatter than any of our other animals because we are, in fact, going to put her down soon. Even though much time has passed and I have since had my own child, I still fight for Number 587 to have one more chance.

My husband keeps saying, "You are a person, she is a cow. You need to get over this." But, I can't. And Number 587 is yet another reason this book needed to be written; not in any weird dedication sort of way but because, through my ridiculous instinct to protect her, I realized that I am just trying to protect myself. I don't want to be viewed like Number 587; worthless because I had a hard time making babies.

Through that revelation, the clouds over my struggle lifted and I finally had a few moments of clarity. It is both stupid of me to feel that way and perfectly acceptable. On the ladder of emotions that pulse through your body during the climb toward parenthood, the rung of feared worthlessness will definitely be one you must overcome. This will only be one of the hundreds of thousands of other emotions that make you thankful others cannot hear your thoughts.

*Journal Entry - Just started IVF #2*
  *I cannot get my thoughts in a manageable order. I want to cry, then scream, then pull my hair out, then eat something sweet, then cry again. I feel worthless and have no pride in myself, though I have several projects that I have accomplished lately that I am quite proud of. See what I mean, I don't make any sense. The worst part is that it only gets more intense from here on out!*

You have never before been through this situation so it is normal to feel things you are not used to feeling. Blame. Fear. Pain. Confusion. Some new emotion you have no name for. It's OK to feel. It's OK to be alone. It's OK to blurt out craziness. It's OK to feel in a big way! Give yourself permission.

You're in survival mode. You have to be sensitive to other people, yes. But ultimately you have to survive. It made me feel better sometimes just to do what I needed to do, even if it was not what I would have done in any other circumstance.

*Journal Entry - Start of IVF #2*
  *First shot. I just woke up and gave it to myself. I did not tell Matt, I just did it all alone. Which is exactly the way I feel. Last time Matt was there for my first couple of shots and towards the end he wanted to give me all of the shots so that he could be involved. I am positive he wants that now too, but I just cannot let him in quite yet.*

I will shamefully admit I fought a great battle with jealousy. Everyone was pregnant and I was not. Again, it is OK to be jealous. Just make sure you manage it. You must realize that you are not being punished. I went through a phase where I was concerned that my fertility curse was a result of punishment for the mistakes I had made in my past. I was not a Christian until I was 21 and I had plenty of time to act without the tightest standards. In fact, since being a Christian, I still do not follow God's path to the scriptural letter 100% of the time. I fall short as every Christ follower does. So, I created the idea that God was getting even.

When speaking to my girlfriends in similar situations, they often tell me the exact same thing - that if they could apologize for their past wrongdoings they would. We discuss how, if we could make some kind of bargaining for future failures, we would do that too. We would do anything to become a mother.

God does not punish me or you for the sheer act of punishing. Though fertility problems do feel like punishment, it is important that you know that is not what is happening.

In fact, God loves you and is allowing this difficulty for some kind of good purpose. He will work it all together for good. Don't roll your eyes.

I walked the Susan G. Komen Breast Cancer Three-Day for the first time in 2002. This is a three day journey that covers sixty miles. My team of four along with 3,000 women and men would painfully walk long distances and up very large hills. In order to keep up the climb, I would say "What goes up...", to which my empowering friend, Whitnie, would loudly reply "...must come down," and together we got through it.

When crossing the finish line, those hills became a large part of our perceived achievement. Our bodies ached but only temporarily. Our backs were sweaty but only for a time. We thought we could not take another step and then we did. We walked all seemingly impossible 60 miles in three days.

The same concept applies to infertility. The hill is steep but our husbands, friends and family will support us until we can comfortably enjoy the downhill glide toward success.

Your body may be weary from shots, pills and potions but it is only temporary and when you are finally called "Mom", you will not even remember the ache.

Your back may not be sweaty but your heart will be overworked from being uplifted with good news and crumbled with bad. Your spirit will beg for love and shun it at the same time. Be strong and take courage knowing that this too shall pass.

When you get to the point where you cannot take another step, please look around and realize that, just by looking, you are moving forward. We often need to grab some perspective to make it through the hike.

Give yourself permission to feel whatever you feel to the fullest degree and then move on. Blame. Hate. Love. Fight. Keep your eye on Jesus and your marriage. It'll be OK.

# SARCASTIC CONGRATULATIONS TO YOU

When it comes to handling baby showers or the big announcement that yet another friend is pregnant, you get pretty good at faking congratulations.

While you are undeniably happy for your friend or family member that God has chosen her to be a mother, you are reminded by way of the announcement that He has not yet chosen you. The pendulum of emotion can be dizzying.

I have made no secret through the writing of this book that I suffered a serious case of jealousy. I can only apologize to myself and those I love for the green monster that manipulated me for such a long period of time.

I once read that jealousy is like taking poison and expecting the other person to die. It is so true that the person who suffers most in this unbalanced emotional state is the one chewing on the jagged pill of envy.

I will be honest, this was the most difficult chapter for me to incorporate in the book. Not because it is the most personal, but because it is the most grotesque. I am ashamed of my behavior and my reaction in the stories I will share with you. However, I feel that in exposing my weakness of character, you will realize that you too are allowed to be imperfect. Please, as you read this chapter forgive me along the way and understand that, with prayer and time, I am now healed just as you one day will be too.

I have several absolutely wonderful girlfriends that I could not live without and I need each of them and their time. I have weekly Bible studies with several of them. I have constant phone calls with a few of them. I email all of them. We even invented the "girlfriend kidnapping."

The first girlfriend kidnapping happened when Laurie and I discovered that we knew a bunch of great girls who did not know each other. So we made a plan to pick them up for dinner and a movie one evening. Instead of calling them and arranging things the normal way, Laurie and I pieced together a ransom note made of magazine clippings for each girl. The words appeared "The lady of the house will be kidnapped (by friends)"... on this date at this time, etc.

It was a huge hit and the group expands and contracts as work gets busy, people move away and babies come. It has been so much fun, but during my fertility-less stint, I couldn't help but retreat from them all. Even my very best friends, in a way, were removed both physically and emotionally a bit from me. I could not tell them the raw and uncensored truth about my emotions on the situation because they were ALL pregnant (or so it seemed in my eyes). And because they were all pregnant, they all had baby showers!

It felt like I was going to one shower or another every weekend for a year. Of course this is a gross over exaggeration, but when the whole entire female population is birthing and you are not, one baby shower on one weekend might as well be 52.

I love those girls and I was so happy for them, but in some way my jealousy of them overshadowed my happiness. I wanted so badly to be pregnant. They were pregnant and I was not and that hurt!

I remember when three of my close friends all got pregnant about the same time. One friend was due in January. She started "trying" around the same time we did – her daughter was three years old before our baby, Sam, was conceived! Another close friend had a baby in February and my business partner had her child in March. Yeah, it made me want to die with envy.

One thing you must know is my mother's nickname for me: Cruise Director. If there is an event to be had, then you have a good bet that I am behind the planning in some way or another. I love parties, gatherings, dinners out, slumber parties, cocktail parties, dinner parties, martini Fridays, fund raisers, wedding showers, bridal luncheons, bachelorette parties, cookouts, cookins and shindigs. I love planning them all, including baby showers, until I was plagued with the I word.

In fact, my next book just may be about creative party ideas. We once were raising money for the Breast Cancer Three-Day, which is the 60-mile, three day walk, fund raiser and awareness builder that I mentioned earlier. Each participant must raise $2,000 before they can walk in this massive event. There were six of us girls heading to Chicago to do this walk and we needed a wingding for a fund raiser. So, we invented "The Boob-B-Q"

It was one of the best parties I have ever hosted. Friends, family and a few strangers paid at my front door to enter and received a sticker that said "I love boobs!" Inside they munched on a menu that included Shish-ka-boobs, tater tatas, melons, jugs of beer, chicken breasts and a boob cake. Seriously, it was a kick! People arrived with flashing light pins stuck to their shirt in just the right place (wink wink), pink boas around their neck and a good time on their face. It was a classic (maybe classless) thematic party!

However, when it came time to throw a bash for my full-bellied girlfriends, I was lame. We did have a double surprise party for the two first due and it was pretty cool, but my "cruise director" self was not fully engrossed in the process. Their pregnancies occurred before my conception woes really reared its ugly head. So I was slightly jealous of them, but not so much so that it blackened my otherwise rosy heart.

Through my four years of wishing, hoping and praying for a healthy pregnancy, my love of parties wavered. Not only did I not want to attend baby showers but I didn't want to attend any party. I was cautious of being around any group that included women of child bearing age. I was trying to manage my emotions, which was super difficult while being hopped up on pharma-created hormones.

As time passed and I remained NOT pregnant, it seemed that my personal worst nightmares were unfolding. None of them are the kind of horror stories that include Freddie Krueger or a Jason mask. These are all wonderful goings-on for the world, but personally deflating for me at the time.

Again, bear with me here. I am opening up to you and sharing some major weaknesses and vulnerabilities. I am putting some of my worst moments and meanest thoughts on display. I am being honest about how I felt in the heat of my raw emotion. I am laying a few instances out there for you. I want you to take them with a grain of salt, knowing I was often hopped up on serious hormone therapy along with a few evil heartbreak and jealousy concoctions that would have killed anything in radius but were instead boiling within me.

So, again, forgive me and read between those lines. I include them so that you can see the real story; so you can have a sense of "permission" to be who you are while also finding someone to relate to in my story; so you can learn from my mistakes and be stronger as you proceed through this ugliness on to hope; so that you can take from these stories what might be beneficial to your friendships in the long run.

## Bible Study Debacle

We have had a weekly Bible study for five years now and I hope that never changes, but during this fertility-challenged time in my life, I was less than eager to attend, though I did anyway. The group was in a transitional time because we had recently lost a couple of members due to pregnancies and newborn babies.

My body was undergoing its own transition and I was barely able to sit on the couch because the fluffiness of it would painfully touch the top part of my progesterone-in-oil injected bottom. Matt and I had found out the week prior to this particular meeting that our first round of IVF was unsuccessful and I was throwing a roaring pity party in my heart.

My girlfriends had been sensitive toward me, afraid to ask how things had gone or how I was feeling. I had just told the group that God did not grant us this child when I noticed one Bible studier turning a little green. She got up and excused herself. Carol's Kermit-the-Frog hue appeared two more times that evening.

Our studies follow a certain format: Get snacks, briefly chat, open in prayer, do the study questions, discuss throughout, then follow with prayer requests and a long prayer. During the prayer request time, we go around the room and discuss those items in our life that we would like to remind God to look after (as if He doesn't already know). We had heard the usual so-and-so is traveling, such and such had surgery, Kristine and Matt want a baby, blah blah blah. Then we get to Carol and her yellowish green color face and she announces... she is pregnant.

This is joyous news and I was truly happy for her. Carol had lost a child about two months into a previous pregnancy and this healthy conception was a blessing. All of that is so true and still, to a woman whose heart has been shattered by yet another failed attempt to procreate, the news felt a great deal like choking on water that went down the wrong way. You don't want to make a big deal because you have been swallowing for 84,000 years and yet you can still mess it up. Nonetheless, you have a choking sensation that does become embarrassing because you know that everyone knows what is going on.

Carol needed not be sensitive to my circumstance. She had fabulous news and it was worthy of praise to God and prayers for a continued healthy development. However, my comfortable Bible study sanctuary, where everyone knew my difficulties, had been lost. Not because of something anyone else had done, but because I outcast myself in my own shame and grief.

This story may not seem like a big deal to some, but when you lose your haven to yet another pregnancy, it is a debilitating blow.

I understand now, that it is common with fertility battles to feel shattered and isolated. It is acceptable to be quiet and introverted (even if it is not in your usual realm of characteristics).

Just plan to give it some time, get your mind right and then call the pregnant person later and tell them the scoop: "I'm so happy for you but when I hear news like this it breaks my heart a little bit more because I can't get pregnant. I'm jealous and I'm sorry I did not show you how wonderfully happy I sincerely am for you." (Make up your own words, but you get the point.) Be honest and that will feel better. You'll make room for yourself to be sensitive in future moments without explanation.

All we ask from those that are pregnant is that you be a little sensitive. Please know your audience and if there is a woman who needs time with the news of your blessing, tell them early.

### Cookout Come Out

At a St. Patrick's Day event at a famous local restaurant, I was visiting with a guy who worked with Matt. His wife is a good friend. He confided in me that they had been trying to get pregnant for a little while. He sought advice from me about the steps we had taken in our procreation battle plan. Matt and I were still fighting the good fight and I was eager to talk about it.

I felt empowered and encouraged that my trials were leading to information for my friends. This conversation was one of the moving cogs, in fact, that led me to write this book.

He and I had a wonderful talk. I never discussed our conversation with my girlfriend. She is a very private person and if she had wanted me to know they were trying to conceive, she would have told me herself. I honestly almost forgot about the St. Patrick's Day conversation with her husband. I forgot, that is, until I started noticing the signs.

Every one of us who are struggling through this 'issue' knows the signs of an impending pregnancy announcement. It is like we are given a kind of super human power to detect additional life within another. It is not a gift we like. We are stuck sulking privately with the knowledge until the announcement is made and then we are forced to fake it just a teensy tiny bit more.

What were the signs? First, my friend's mom owns a liquor store so she is constantly bringing a bottle of wine for the host of any gathering. She had stopped making that gesture. Then I began to notice at social functions that she never, ever drank anything with alcohol and avoided caffeine too. The final straw to break the camel's back was the extra pound or two. She is an absolutely beautiful, tall, slender, little thing, so extra pounds are very noticeable on her frame.

Some months down the road, we were at a co-workers home for a backyard bar-b-que. I had had enough of this "is-she-pregnant-ness" and I wanted to know for sure. So I simply asked her hubby the question "when is she due?" He looked at me with the how-much-do-you-know look and I just smiled.

He told me she was about four months along but did not want anyone to know until she worked up the courage to tell her employer. It turns out that even when he and I were having our St. Patrick's Day discussion, she was already pregnant but did not know it yet. I smiled and congratulated him. I told him that I would not share this new knowledge until she was ready to tell me.

I held that congratulatory mask up to my face just long enough to excuse myself and slip around the corner of the house. I remember looking up at the sky and being thankful to see the darkening clouds, as if God knew I was going to need a cover for my tears and wanted to cry with me. I climbed into our parked car and melted into a sadness that was unlike anything I had ever felt before. Come to think of it, this must have been just before our IVF failure because my poor body was covered with needle marks from the hormones.

So, what does a girl do when she is in so much emotional pain she literally can't see through her tears? Everyone handles those times differently, but this girl calls her best friend. Yep, I called Laurie immediately. All my sweet Laurie could do was listen and apologize for not being right beside me. And, really, that is all she could do. No words make it feel better and no words really should.

Again, I love this now pregnant girlfriend and I was extremely happy (somewhere in my heart) for their good news. Even so, for those initial moments and days, all I could see was that she was experiencing what I could not have... what I may never have. I had thought she was going to share my pain of a slowed fertility and I could somehow mentor her through that, which might make my pain somehow feel more worth it. Instead, there she sat with one button of her jeans undone from her expanding belly.

As I look back, I can see that misery must certainly love company. I did not and do not wish the kind of problems about ourselves and our situation we had on anyone. But honestly, there was comfort in the conversation I had with my friend's husband because it let me know I was not solitary. Before my conversation with him, I had not considered the fact that other women were experiencing this same difficulty. We have a natural tendency to think we are all alone in our hardships and that not another soul on this earth has experienced what we have. That's when, somehow, there's comfort in the "I'm NOT that special" lesson of earlier.

This is part of my journal entry from the day following the party where I learned of her pregnancy.

*Journal Entry*
*The deal is, I knew this was coming and yet I still cannot deal with it. I try to mentally prepare myself for these kinds of things but I am incapable. I knew that at our last Bible study meeting, the first one in the series with the book "A Mary Heart in a Martha World," that I would be confronted with several baby issues. Carol is pregnant, as is Kim. But I was not ready to discuss how wonderful and precious it is and how everyone knows someone who just had a baby, is about to have a baby, is surprisingly expecting or wishes they were not pregnant. It was deflating! I felt like jumping up with a neon signs that read "Have mercy, I cannot take this and you are being very inconsiderate of me here!"*

*True, I have had a White Russian (I am not pregnant and so I can have a little somethin' somethin' every once in a while). Plus, I am about to start my period, but I have a right to feel this way. I have big fat lost something and this is not fair! I hate the word "fair" but I am giving myself permission to feel that this situation sucks and it is not fair. I pray, pray, pray that God has something fantastic planned from all of this because that is the only thread tying me to reality. Seriously, the only one.*

Hindsight being 20/20, I should have come up with the proper mindset and a phrase or two of response. I should have looked at myself in the mirror weeks ago and said "Kristine, if anyone tells you they are pregnant, say 'That is fantastic news. You two will make brilliant parents.'" Then rehearse that over and over until it becomes real. People around you WILL get pregnant, just be prepared.

My friend and her husband did nothing wrong. There is not a single thing that should have been done differently. This story was a propagation of my instability.

## The Big Ouch!

My experience with Lindsay was by far the most difficult of them all. She and I became friends through a professional development program that is geared towards creating community leaders by educating them as to the inner workings and needs that surround our town. We were the youngest in the group, which seemed to be status quo for the two of us; both intelligent, ambitious go-getters who love to rapidly communicate and get the proverbial ball rolling in any situation. We were designed to be friends and that was clear from our earliest interactions.

We had so much in common. We live in a small college town, where most people become educated and then move away. This leaves people like us with great friends who live great distances away. We were both married with no children and had almost zero local friends. So, we latched onto each other like a sucker fish to the side of a tank.

While getting to know Lindsay better, I learned how very much she wanted to be a career woman. Children would come, she hoped, but not for a very long time. Questions about her marriage loomed in her mind. She wanted a career before kids for sure, or at least that was the plan she was creating for herself. Have you ever seen the bumper sticker "If you want to make God laugh, tell him your plans?" That turned out to be the case with her.

A few months into our friendship, she told me that she wasn't feeling quite right. "You're pregnant," I told her. She would not hear it. She was on birth control and a person on birth control cannot possibly get pregnant.

Her career was on the move and she'd just started a new job. Finally, concerned about the fact that she'd be traveling and her periods were irregular, she decided to see the doctor. The phone nurse advised that they'd probably just change her pill's prescription since she'd been on it a while. They changed it alright – to a prenatal vitamin!

That's right! Her baby was conceived while she was on birth control. She had three periods while pregnant, although they were late and unusual. So, by the time she went to the doctor, she was 12 weeks along. She and her husband were having a baby in just six months and they had no idea!

She had a hard time adjusting to the idea of rearranging her professional goals, but this ended up being the very best thing in the whole wide world. Her son is amazing and God knew right when to make him.

We are getting to the "ouch," just hang tight.

As I told you earlier, Matt and I had decided when the time came to try to have kids, we'd pull a certain bottle of wine from the rack and that would be the last day I'd take my pill. So, about two months before Lindsay's baby was due, Matt and I popped the cork to that South African bottle of wine and decided to become parents.

Lindsay was very much aware of our dream to conceive and was there every month to hear about how I had seen red in the potty again. She was there when I started Clomid and heard that my eggs were too small. She had intimate knowledge of our frustration at the slowness of conception and had been a loyal friend every step of the way.

When her son was one, we were invited to his birthday party. Yes, I'd be attending a big birthday bash, still with no baby in my belly. The whole family was in attendance including a few good friends. Lindsay called and asked me to come a few minutes early, so I arrived with five minutes to spare just to help out. Upon arrival and hellos, she swept me off where we could be alone and said "I have to tell you something." I was clueless, but I humored her. "I'm having a baby," she nervously announced to me.

She started to cry. She handed me a photo of the ultrasound and told me that they were about to tell the whole family but needed me to know first. She told me that she was using birth control again and still got pregnant…that she was already four months along so her children would obviously be very close together in age.

I was stunned. I hugged her in congratulations and smiled. We left the room and busied ourselves with the party. I smiled at people a few more times until I could find Matt. I grabbed the arm of my husband and told him we had to leave. The pale Casper-like color of my face told him there was no discussion in the matter.

We sat in the parked car and I told him the whole story. He encouraged me that things were going to be fine. He said that we should march right back into that birthday party with our smiles on because "Lindsay is your friend and you need to support her." My husband is annoyingly right about things like this.

During the party, the announcement was made. It was a neat moment for their families. Then it hit me.

My friend was four months pregnant and did not tell me! She later assured me that not telling me was just because her own shock and emotion didn't allow her to verbalize it to anyone. To me, it felt like she had intentionally kept this enormous secret from me to spare my emotions. I imagined that, in trying to protect me, she hurt me in ways only a woman could know. She admitted that pain for me was part of her difficulty in accepting her own pregnancy.

That was it. It was time to go. Enough birthday surprises for me. When we got to the car I doubled over with nausea. Nothing came out except tears. In the midst of all my struggles, I really have to be close to someone who gets pregnant with birth control miracle babies.

The first two crushing moments were functions of my own emotional weaknesses. This one, which came before the others, was because I felt managed. I felt like she did not want to hurt me by revealing the news so she kept it a secret. I now know that wasn't the reason for her secretive behavior, but feeling manipulated and pitied was a harsh slap in the face.

Thankfully, I was not to the high point of my selfish jealousy, so this event did not take the toll it could have if it had happened 12 months later. But it did happen with this close, close friend and that is where the greatest sting occurred.

This story is yet another reason I felt this book had to be written. She felt the pangs of pregnancy in the opposite way I did, with fear and concern of the speed and timing God had created. Hers would be a book I would love to read. She says "we learned parallel lessons on perpendicular planes. We both learned that God is in charge and we can't change things." Parallel lessons, yes, but there are parts of the story that the other will never relate to no matter how hard we try.

The good news is that we are still close today. We stayed committed. We hung in there and communicated. I love her and those precious little miracle babies and she loves me and my precious little miracle babies. Being infertile doesn't give you a pass to behave like a jerk. Likewise, being super-fertile doesn't give you a pass to be overly sensitive to the point unintentionally of hurting someone.

My mind did the right thing by not processing all that was going on at one time. By not realizing (until I took part in her moment) that she had kept a big fat secret from me for months, I was able to shut my otherwise very open mouth. I recommend doing the same when you are posed under similar circumstances. Also, I allowed myself the ability to leave early. Do that if you need to. Real friends always understand.

It is important to understand that this was our most strenuous friendship period. But fortunately, friendship is elastic and it can come back together. You can mess it all up and then work it all out.

## Scream

Claire has been married for several years. They are happy in their marriage. They are both healthy and active. She is an intellectual. He laughs at everything – especially movie lines. They are a stable and amazing couple who has been trying for quite some time to get pregnant. Together, they will make excellent parents.

But, instead of Claire getting pregnant, her older, less stable, single sister gets pregnant. If you want to know what it feels like to be shot in the lungs without a gun being fired I would say the day Claire learned this news was about as close as you are going to get.

As we can imagine, Claire was happy her sister was going to bring new life into the world and that she would have a nephew to love. But, damn it! An unmarried bar tender who didn't expect a baby versus her married, stable sister who is anxiously awaiting that moment – it was a tough pill to swallow.

The peak of difficulty, or at least what I was privy to know about, was her sister's baby shower. Claire is never late to an event. In fact, she is usually early and prepared to help you set out the chips and welcome the rest of the gang. For this event, however, her car just could not reach its destination.

She called me several minutes after the party began and told me she was fifteen minutes away. Claire wanted to support her sister, but she just could not find the strength to pull herself together.

I did what any friend who really knows her pain would do. I cried with her over the phone. She was in the driver's seat of her Toyota on the way to the shower and I was sitting on my unmade bed at home and we, together, screamed as loud and as long as our lungs would allow. I highly recommend this stress relieving tactic. Get vocal!

Scream your head off if you need to. It is a wonderful band-aid! If you are lucky enough to have a friend that will cry with you without even having to explain the details, call them often.

I believe that Claire's sister gave her some grace and temporarily lowered her expectation level so that Claire could get her heart, mind and spirit back in balance without making a forever relationship-damaging mistake in the heat of fury. Other than not getting pregnant first, this is the best thing her sister could have done.

I know, oh so well, that showers and pregnancy announcements are a special kind of torture. These are your friends and you really should not bow out when it comes to sharing their joy. These people love you and you love them and you must not lose site of the bigger picture. You are perfectly allowed to be selective in the invitations you choose to accept. If she is not a close pal, then you can send a gift and your well wishes with another friend. Don't feel guilty if you need to do this for yourself. Later, when you are more stable and able to communicate to that friend, you can tell her the truth if you want to. When I did this with my friends, they perfectly understood and would have had it no other way. No buddy of yours will want her happiness to cause you pain. Ninety percent of the time, they will get it.

If you do happen to attend a shower, I have also found that a huge helper is chatting with other non-parents. They are fairly easy to spot. They are the women with manicured hair and nothing wet and clumpy on the shoulder of their shirt. This will give you things to talk about such as work, who you both know at the shower, blah blah blah.

Another sneaky trick for removing weight from your emotional baggage is to shop for showers at Wal-Mart or Target or some other general store that is not Babies-Only. These all-baby-all-the-time shops can do a number on your heart. Those cute little pink and blue onsies will melt you heart and then break it again. Just don't put yourself through that if you can help it. And if you must, make sure there's an unrelated department nearby for your breather.

As noted in the "Prepare Yourself" section of the Advice chapter, you need to... well... prepare yourself. Don't let your personal dilemma create more drama between you and the friends you love dearly. Give them your congratulations, as temporarily sarcastic as it may be...

... and then go on with life.

# WAITING IS THE WORST

$\mathcal{W}$aiting is painful. Can I get an "Amen!"? It is the worst part of the entire battle. Shots are torture, no question, but they are active. You are physically engaged as you move one prick closer to a healthy baby.

Don't get me wrong, the previous chapter is not void now. Showers and announcements are excruciatingly painful, but they are comparable to ripping off the band aid. There are just so many steps in the battle with fertility that include not doing a cotton-picking thing... except waiting and I personally believe that to be the worst kind of torture.

Here is THE sentence we all hate the very most. "Just give it time."

Shut up already! Time has already been given. I have given it time, I have waited enough. Do I sound angry? Then you must be the friend reading this. Anyone who's gone through infertility or is going through it knows exactly what this is like. I'm not normally angry, but inactively waiting is too much to handle!

Let's say you go to the doctor and he tells you to try a medication like Clomid, for example. You take the pills and then you wait for them to work and wait for your next appointment. Then you wait to see an ultrasound to know if your eggs are larger or if there are more of them. Basically, you swallow then sit on your behind twiddling your thumbs.

If you have chosen to wait one more month to see if your period comes, that is another hair-pulling 28-30 days. Yes, there is sex in there, but by this time even that can begin to feel like a chore instead of a passionate embrace of lovers.

The off-the-charts most torture-filled waiting comes after you have had some kind of process done like IUI (Intra-Uterine Insemination) or IVF (In Vitro Fertilization) or one of the other 84,000 three-letter acronyms meant to describe eggs and sperm meeting in some fancy (and expensive) way.

After my IVF treatments, I was instructed to lie in bed for three days with no activity other than going to the bathroom. I remember looking at my tummy and praying with an intensity I hadn't known before. I remember stepping into my shower and looking down thinking "my belly looks a little bit fuller, maybe it worked." Of course your body does not respond that quickly, but I was sure that I knew my body so well that I could tell if I was five days pregnant. While wadding up the toilet paper every time I would go to the bathroom, I found myself kind of chanting "please don't see red, please don't see red, please don't see red."

Lighthearted side note - My friend, Gina and I have had some very long and interesting conversations about the proper way to use toilet paper. She and I are of the habit of unrolling the paper off the holder (from the top of course, if it comes from underneath then it is backwards) and making a wad. We have found that many of our male friends, husbands included, are folders. She and I have come to the determination that since we, as women, use the paper far more frequently, then we must be doing it the most effective and least time consuming way. I have one female friend who says she is a roller. Something about taking it from the cardboard roll stuck to the wall and rolling it on your hand, then taking it off her hand and voila. This makes no sense to me at all. The way she described it makes me think more of a mitt than a roll. Anyway, you will be surprised how adamant people are about their toilet paper style. Changing to a different method after you're set in your ways is pretty much impossible. If you have comments about this, I'll get you Gina's contact information because she is the one who started it! She is also the one who started the debate over defining the phrase "making out". I say it is just kissing and she says it is much, much more. Gina and I were college roommates, which is to say we had a lot of valuable time spent talking about invaluable things.

Back to the waiting. (Did I mention that, while waiting, it's good to reminisce and let your mind wander to random things like college roommate conversations and toilet paper?) Oh, yea, back to the waiting. All of these little steps of waiting are painful, there is no doubt. However, it is the overwhelming collaboration of them all that makes fertility problems so difficult to manage on a daily basis.

*Journal Entry*

*Our whole state is covered in ice so my medication will arrive by UPS tomorrow sometime between 8 and 3. Don't you just love how they give you those windows of action that might as well be "sometime between January and April"? Fortunately (or unfortunately), Matt is sick so he will stay home tomorrow and accept the package and I can run my errands and keep this off my mind. As if.*

*Journal Entry*

*The nurse wanted me to increase the dose of my Repronex shot. Note this journal entry is a flashback, therefore, not written on the day in question. As it turns out I screwed up my medication big time and my fit of crying and freaking out did not allow me to write yesterday.*

*Here is the deal. I am supposed to take five powders tonight. Matt gives me the shots, therefore, I have been relatively unaware of the quantities of medication I have had remaining. I thought I had four powders left when in fact I had none. I was sure that this was the end of the process as well as life as I knew it. Not only could I not have a baby but I can't even keep track of my meds! This further proves that God does not want me to have a baby. I bawled my eyes out to the point of almost throwing up. The kind of crying that is miserable on the crier and anyone within a three-mile radius who does not have a canoe for safety.*

*Obviously, I would need more Repronex and had to find a pharmacy that could supply me. It is important to note that when I realized I did not have enough medication it was about 5:30 p.m.. Luck not being on my side, I could not find the phone book in this entire house and I promise you I turned it upside down. You would have thought a loved one had passed away with my behavior. I was uncontrollable.*

*Once mildly composed I turned to our ever reliable Internet to give me the phone numbers of local pharmacies. Yeah... the computer was "frozen" and would not work. Again I commenced the freaking out.*

*If you are not a college sports fan, you will not get this part, but to compound the trauma to my already miserable heart, I could not find the Oklahoma State vs. Kansas State basketball game on TV. See, I had tickets to this game which started at 6:00 but since only 30 minutes prior I went stark raving mad, there was no way I was going to make an appearance at Gallagher-Iba Arena.*

*Let me recap: I can't find the basketball game on TV, the phone book is missing, the computer is broken, I have no medication, I am fairly certain the whole expensive, painful process is shot and we have not yet accomplished world peace. To a man this list seems random and nothing worth crying two hours over. To any over estrogen-ized woman, hysteria makes perfect sense.*

*There are no pharmacies in town that carry the prescribed medication. Not a huge shocker since I currently order the stuff from New Jersey. I call the "on-call" nurse several times for advice and remedy. To make an already long story short, she outlined a plan to save the process so I wouldn't have to wait and start the med cycle all over again. The nurse's calm voice and firm action plan (plus a call with Laurie) had me soothed as much as possible.*

*I should mention that I received constant text messages on my phone from Matt about love and the game's score. I made him go to the game without me since I would not wish the wrath of my emotions on anyone.*

This long journal entry was not weirdly placed. Keep following me.

I often pray for patience. I have decided that God is granting me this wish by way of infertility and thus teaching me this lesson in a large way. I once heard "be careful for what you wish for... it may come true." Instead of the lesson for patience, perhaps I should have asked for enlightenment. Getting patience is not really that fun.

These journal entries are very personal, thus, I share them with the entire world. See what I mean in the advice chapter about being afraid that the whole world will roll their eyes at my intense pity party?

But, sharing this uncensored moment helps me hammer in my point. If you are going through your own personal fertility nightmare, you are waiting on something. It may be your medication, it may be your period, it may be your test results, it may be for your husband to come around to aggressive measures you are willing to take in order to create your family. It does not matter what you are waiting for, because we are all waiting to create the family we know we should have.

One of the most difficult aspects of the waiting game is not the treatments or the outcome, but the hold it puts on life. I used to own a very small but mildly successful graphic design and advertising firm. It was not much, but it kept a full time salary for me, my partner and a few part timers. I decided to sell my share of the company when I entered into the IVF program. I knew I would frequently visit specialists in a bigger city with an hour commute and that my hormones and emotions would, in no way, allow me to be professional. I also knew I wanted to stay home when my eventual family came. The time was right, but the decision was still difficult. I sold my business… and then had a failed attempt of pregnancy. Talk about a blow!

My career was in a state of shock. What the hell do I do now? I questioned everything. Every single one of my decisions turned to ash. I felt like I could not plan for the future at all.

Another one of my friends is going through her own fertility-less void. She has to plan her work schedule a month in advance. As women who are experiencing fertility treatments all know, we are on the schedule our body creates. It is not ours for juggling. Like clockwork, every month when her supervisor asks her when she needs off, she has to relive the feeling of waiting on her body. She also moonlights as a consultant for a company that requires travel to other states. That company is constantly asking her for months of planning and she can't comply.

If you have a salaried position that does not require a changing schedule, travel, or clocked in hours, then you are lucky. If your treating physician is in the same town and easily accessible, then you are even more lucky (relatively speaking, of course). If this employer also provides health insurance that covers infertility, then you have won the lottery. That is not the case for so many.

It is difficult to balance between being a solid, steady employee and a flaky member of the staff with erratic behaviors. It really does feel like everything is on hold: the project you are working on, the career goals you have outlined, quitting all together to stay at home with the kids you so desperately want.

I was begging God for some kind of sign. "What should I do and when. Please God, I need direction. I don't know what to do!"

This is going to sound sappy as hell, so if you are not in that mood, then skip this last part and move on to the following chapter.

Waiting is never going to feel good. But, take solace in the truth that waiting evolves into an opportunity for self-exploration, spiritual development and relationship building. The journal entry about patience was very gratifying because I realized something invaluable: this experience has a purpose. I learned a great deal about myself and I found unbreakable strength in my marriage. I learned that God really is in control of the universe (regardless of how very much I would like to give it a try). Therefore, I recommend you journal, share your feelings and emotions, get introspective, busy yourself with worthwhile distractions and then cycle back through all of those things.

When your life changes and you are given the news that you will be a parent, magically the past months and years of struggle and disappointment will vanish from memory. That time becomes your badge of honor and, while you may not wear it proudly, you undeniably wear it in terms of your changed behavior and attitude.

I had a great discussion with my friend just the other evening. She was telling me how difficult this process has been and how she finds herself just praying and praying and praying for some kind of resolve and that is when it hit me. Maybe the struggle of waiting is God's way of bringing her closer to Him. I know that is exactly what happened for me.

I begged God hourly for a family. I prayed and thought about the situation constantly. One day I went to church with Matt and we began the book of Samuel. The book opens with Hannah crying and begging God for a child. I related to her instantly. One day she went to the temple in such a state that the priest thought she was drunk. Finally he realized that she was inconsolably distraught and he told her that her prayer for a child would be answered by God. It was. Hannah had a baby boy and "she named him Samuel because she asked him of the Lord." (1 Sam 1:20) I left church that day knowing that if I was given the gift of a baby boy, I too would name him Samuel. Samuel Matthew is the light of my life today. Stay patient in your waiting.

# Patiently Waiting

Baby, I love you, though God has not yet given you to me;
I spend my whole life learning patience and that is now what I am trying to be.


I love you though we have not met, and though you are not yet real;
Somehow you are in every thought, and love is all I feel.


You're a dream I didn't know I had, a prayer I didn't know I would pray;
A song that I would sing to you, if only you would stay.


We want you in our life to share a love that is so strong;
And we will continue to wait for you - it does not matter how long.


We believe God's perfect plan so you will come when the time is right;
And though you are not real yet, you are already Mommy's delight.


I want to hold you in my arms and teach you to be great;
I want you to be our legacy, our destiny, our fate.


Your daddy and I love you and we can't wait for the day;
When we can kiss you gently and you will not go away.


We have a wonderful marriage, maybe this hardship is our test;
But holding hands together, we continue to pray for the best.


That you will grace our lives with greatness and make us a family;
So the love that is too much for two can soon be shared by three.

# Chapter Eleven

# MELTING YOUR MASK

$\mathcal{T}$housands of years have passed since the Bible was first written. History and cultural changes make parts of the Bible and its vocabulary seem, well, weird. I revealed in the chapter about marriage relationships that I used to despise the word "submit." As in "wives you will submit to your husbands." Now that I understand the meaning and context of the word, it is not so frightening. In fact, I now find great personal strength in being the kind of wife that biblically submits to my husband who is also submitting to God and loving me with his whole heart.

Before becoming a believer, I was closed-hearted to understanding what I read in the bible. On the rare occasion that I did read it, the Bible didn't make a lick of sense to me. I also did not read it for education and understanding. Instead I hunted for morsels of scripture I could use in a debate against the King. Now that I've studied it for years and listened to teachers who help me put the historical, cultural and Symantec details in the right perspective, the Bible has blossomed into a simple and comforting instruction book for living life.

Sometimes the way of a women reminds me of my Bible reading

evolution. Unintentionally we women speak in clips of speech so that only those who really know us understand what we are saying.

When you ask a woman about children and she responds with something to the effect of "we are not trying but we are not trying to stop it either," that is code for "we really want a baby and have stopped using contraception. I know exactly when my cycle ends and begins and what goes on in the middle but I don't want you to pressure me with questions about it yet."

There are thousands of codes that can only truly be decoded when you have experienced the situation with an open heart.

A buddy had sent out an email pleading for prayers for her second round of Clomid. The email said:

> *I am sending out an email asking for a huge favor. I need some serious prayers this week. As many of you know, we are having fertility problems. We are on our second round of Clomid and I am asking you to pray this week, I know that this is very personal but I need all the help I can get. So, please pray that the Lord will prepare my body, keep me patient and understanding of the situation and allow for us to be supportive to one another throughout the process. If you have prayer groups out there, add us to the list. We need some assistance from the Man up above... Thank you and I know that the Lord will work in His timing. It is just hard to be patient.*

Can you sense the desperation? Don't you just know her pain? If you watched me read this for the first time, you would see streaming tears. It takes a big need for a woman to ask for this kind of help. Surprisingly, this email boosted another friend to ask for the same prayers.

Upon sharing the details of her struggle, I told friend "B" I was glad she was seeking the support I was sure she needed. She countered with "I do need the support but I don't want people asking me about it all the time and adding pressure. I couldn't decide if the support was worth all the questions."

She also noted that, since her decision to tell their secret, couples with similar problems have come out of the woodwork.

See, she had a code. She only wanted people to share in the eventual joy of a pregnancy. She did not want them to know all the battles and struggles that they endured to get to that joy. She masked her true desire, her real emotions.

I look back on the last several months of our friendship and I think of all the times I wish I had known. The times I could have given her the nod of understanding when someone else announced her pregnancy. I think of how I should have known she was waging her own war when she would request a prayer for the 17 friends she had that were pregnant or just had a child and how every week that number went up. That was a blatant sign. You don't count the number of people who are pregnant unless you wish like hell you were one of them.

It is easy to relate to her story. We live in a society where divulging the gift of pregnancy is done in a romantic way. We don't want that tainted by the extended time line, the medication and the shots.

If you are like my friend and don't want people to know of your fight for a family, you are completely entitled. I am a big mouth about everything and shared with every single one of my 84,000 friends and family members that we had popped the wine cork. So when my belly was still relatively flat after a year plus, there was not a lot to discuss.

But if you don't have "diarrhea of the mouth" like me, then I pray that you have one person to be real in front of; one person that can help you carry this load; one soul that knows what you look like without your mask on; and one heart that will break with you because they love you that much.

If that person is your spouse, great. Though, I recommend a girlfriend also. There is something about the shared understanding of another woman that men will just never get. We have a way of knowing when to slap a stamp on a ridiculous card and send it snail mail so that you know we "get it."

Taking off that mask is difficult. More than difficult, it's painful. It's admitting you have a problem. For people in AA, that's the first step. It's our first step too.

Sometimes getting hung up on the terminology and science of it all is a great place to begin taking off the mask. Our society treats us as though we should know everything instantly – thank God for Google. When Matt and I admitted we had a problem, we sought medical advice. I was then finally able to ask the big questions and not feel judged by the doctor or nurse. It was so nice to know that they deal with fertility problems on a daily basis. The problem was, I did not know enough to even ask the right questions. I showed just how ignorant I was fairly quickly.

*Journal Entry*
  *I called the doctor's office about my painful breasts and other yucky stuff. I should have called the fertility clinic but I have asked them some pretty stupid questions in the past and I am a little embarrassed. For example, once I called to ask how many testosterone shots I had to take and the phone nurse said "none, you have to take progesterone, didn't you go to the class?" I feel like an imbecile.*

Sometimes taking off your mask is scary! Do it anyway. It can be a far scarier place if you let yourself dwell in your unhappiness alone with the mask on. This is an extremely personal journal entry and one of those that I wish we did not have to share. Though, I really think you need to know that I do understand what you are going through. Depression, loneliness and ache are common side effects to those of us in this situation. I hope sharing this makes you feel as though you are not solitary in your emotions.

*Journal Entry*

*I know these feelings are medically enhanced, but they are kind of scary. I am unbalanced. I don't like the way I feel about my circumstances, my friends, my life or myself. I want to turn into a hermit and hide from the world. My joy in life has always been to give of myself to others. I love charity and I love to organize events where my friends are all together.*

*Now, however, I don't want to see anyone or do anything. I am so afraid of how situations will make me feel and how I will react. I am scared someone will announce a pregnancy and I will slap them in the face or will share that they lost five pounds and I will feel fat or that they just read a good book and I will think "oh please, like you know how to read."*

*My positive energy has evaporated and what little is left is used for putting on my social mask of normalcy. It takes a great deal of energy to ensure everyone else that I am doing just fine.*

*I give and give to my friends and now I need to be given to. I am lost and sad and I need someone to shelter me with their wings the way I always do for them. You would think that the people who know me best would see these signs and react. But apparently I am such a good actress that they think my decisions and words are legitimate. For example, I quit the Bible study. This is a group that has always been very important to me; a group I started and have led for well over a year now. And I just quit. The reason is that everyone is pregnant and I hate them for it (not literally but I am jealous!). That is only a half truth. I really want to just curl up into a ball in a dark corner and stay there until this is over and my life is back to normal. I wish so much that someone would recognize this and help me out of it.*

My mask was a good one. Yes, I told the world we were having problems with conception, but they did not know much more than that. They did not know the dark destinations I was visiting in my mind. They did not know I needed their support and I was too wrapped up in my own self-pity to ask for help.

There is a commercial for some depression pill that shows a silly cartoon egg going down the road of life. The egg gets sad and loses interest in the things it loved doing before. I was very much that little cartoon egg. Only that egg sought help. So often we women do not. The mask can be a dangerous thing and if it is not dangerous, then it is at least uncomfortable. We need to work at taking it off. This is not to say we need to walk around like zombies with mascara running down our cheeks and a forlorn demeanor, but we need to be true to ourselves.

That mask can be any number of things. It can be not admitting to anyone that you want children. It can be concealing that you have been on fertility meds. It can be concealing your emotional distress. It can even be giving half truths to friends and family when they ask about your baby-making situation or plans. There are hundreds of masks that can be worn and hundreds of reasons for wearing them. My advice is only that you are careful with yourself when it comes to the wearing of these masks. I pray that you know yourself well enough to know when you need to melt that mask and be real.

# Chapter Twelve

# IT'S NOT @#&*ING FAIR!!!

There are a lot of things in this world that aren't fair. Cancer is not fair. War is not fair. Poverty and high-heeled shoes and second-hand smoke are not fair. Tsunamis aren't fair. Telling your four-year-old daughter they lost a soccer game is not fair. Being cheated on by your first boyfriend is not fair and neither are panty hose. Passing out at your wedding is not fair (trust me on this one). Getting tripped up in a race is not fair and neither is your computer crashing in the middle of your term paper. Even sharing is usually not fair.

But when you want a child and the whole wide world is pregnant and you are not, that is a unique kind of not fair (if only because I said so!).

Our first round of IVF did not work. My heart was broken, but my head was held high. If you didn't know we had suffered that loss, you would never have guessed it (mask!). Regardless, we went to church that Sunday following.

We walked in to the church and began our worship. The first song we sang, *Blessed Be Your Name*, brought me to falling tears. It goes like this:

> Every blessing you pour out I'll turn back to praise.
> When the darkness closes in, Lord, still I will say:
> Blessed be the name of the Lord
> Blessed be Your name, Jesus.
> Blessed be the name of the Lord
> Blessed be Your glorious name
> You give and take away
> You give and take away
> My heart will choose to say, Lord, Blessed be your name.

You give and take away?! Can you imagine my tears? I had finally been pregnant but it was taken away. Then this song reminded me that it is God's plan, not mine, that we are living in. Only He knows the outcome.

As I was telling my deep and wonderfully introspective friend, Laurie, I was writing a chapter about things not being fair, she reminded me that grace isn't fair. "We didn't earn our life's blessings and ultimately heaven," she said. "God's grace isn't fair... and thank God that it isn't or we would be hopeless and bound for a meaningless destiny."

Yeah, that is definitely true. Grace is not fair and I praise the Lord for it. While I see her point that grace saves us, it's at a time like this, that grace feels like a cold, drafty room. It should give me comfort that God made things unfair for the reason of giving us wonderful gifts that we don't deserve. The unfairness of it all bruises my soul when it works in the opposite direction. I know this is not punishment or torture, though it really does feel like that.

*Journal Entry*
> *It has been eleven days since I last wrote. The deal is, I have been too emotional to write. I am so confused about feelings, future, etc. that I don't know where to start. So how about I tell you about the*

*last 11 days...*

*We went in on Saturday for the transfer, completely full of life, excitement, optimism and prayers. We get to the clinic, I get changed into basically a sheet and Matt puts on scrubs. We are taking photographs, goofing around and playing because after this day we will be parents, we are so excited. Then the technician walked in and our demeanor changed. She had a serious and very somber look on her face. She took a while to collect her thoughts and then began to cry a little. She told us that there were no thriving or even very viable embryos.*

*I asked if it was even worth doing a transfer and she absorbed the whole room in her long pause. Matt interrupted the loud silence by telling us that "yes it is worth it, those eggs are going to do a lot better inside their mommy."*

*The decision was made to put three eggs in. The one that was late to fertilize looks like a 12-15 cell egg (they want them to be between 32 and 64 cell on transfer day.) They also decided to put two 8-cell eggs in. The technician and the doctor both moved our chances from 65% to around 20-25%. I cried a bit and then decided that would not help matters. If they were putting my babies into my body I was going to be strong for them and for my husband.*

*For the next three days, I laid flat on my back which was apropos, since that is exactly how I felt. It is surprising how taxing that can be on your body. By the middle of day one, my lower back was killing me and nothing but a heating pad and some good old fashioned whining helped. I prayed a lot. I spent tons of time in the presence of God asking for both a miracle and His will to be done. Hoping beyond hope that the two were the same.*

*We recently read a story in church about Jonathan, the son of Saul. Jonathan was to fight the Philistines but God wanted the people of Israel to know He was the one winning the battle. So Jonathan gathered the army together and God narrowed them down in a series of cuts to about 300 men. The Philistines had a huge army and everyone thought Jonathan was crazy for minimizing his soldiers. Of course, God's army did win. My thoughts on this are that sometimes God narrows your chances to prove to you that He is the one winning.*

*This story gave me great comfort and I have told it to many people who try to comfort me when, really, only God can do that. I am not sure what I will do with this lesson should the result of our transfer be negative. Maybe God lowers the chances to show me this is not His way. Though, I am not ready to go down that path yet.*

*So I have been eating a hope sandwich filled with denial and fear and a heaping side of uncertainty. I have been taking my shots every night at 9 p.m. followed by five minutes of butt rubbing and ten minutes of heating pad. It is not nearly as bad as I thought it would be. I just want to milk the sympathy for all it is worth.*

*Saturday I started to have bad pains in my right side even with my hip bone about two inches in. I thought maybe it was appendicitis but with all the shots, stress and abnormal happenings in my belly I knew not to overact. It did not wake me up in the night so I figured it was no big deal. That morning I woke up, went to the restroom and there was a lot of yuckiness. I knew this was not a good sign.*

*I called the fertility clinic a few seconds ago and asked if it was even worth my coming in for the pregnancy test. They said of course it was. So, when Matt gets back from Memphis tomorrow about noon we will head over there to get the final determination.*

*It is amazing what a week of not knowing a life changing and emotionally charged event will do to a person. Had we been able to know on, say, Wednesday, I would have been a total mess either way. I have worked hard at composing myself and doing what Matt calls "mentally preparing." I do not expect the doctor to give us a good diagnosis tomorrow but I do believe in the Lord and his miracles.*

You know the end of this story. Our news was not good because we were not pregnant. The Lord "gives and takes away." In this case, He took away.

This was NOT FAIR!

I did not read C.S. Lewis's book, *The Problem of Pain*. But in Jill Briscoe's book, *Eight Choices That Will Change a Woman's Life*, Jill told me that Lewis wrote: "God whispers to us in our pleasures, speaks in our conscience, but shouts in our pains; it is his megaphone to rouse a deaf world." Wow!

I am pretty sure that nothing earthly gets you through times like this. There is a reason that most people find God in the throes of devastation and difficulty. It is not because He is any more there than He was prior to the situation. It is just that you are more willing to find Him.

Don't get me wrong. I needed Nicole to get me dressed and take me out to lunch. I needed Laurie to send me a cheesy and poignant card. And... I needed chocolate. There is no doubt these things greatly assisted in the process of getting over it.

Even now, as I write these words with my child napping in the other room, I am still devastated by the experience. It has turned into a badge I wear with pride, kind of like a "cancer survivor" button but, like cancer, you don't ever forget the battle.

*Journal Entry*
   *This isn't fair. This isn't fair. This isn't fair.*

   *Please know that as I write this I know that one way or another I will be a mother one day and my husband will be a wonderful father. But right now I cannot hide this emotion from myself anymore than the Sears Tower can hide in the City.*

   *I also know that I will probably get over this feeling. I will probably read this one day and laugh at myself for being so silly. As for today, my heart is absolutely broken and I think this is completely unfair!*

The unfairness will only diminish with the success you will eventually have. I promise, one way or another, you will have success in becoming a parent if you want it badly enough. Until that time, however, you are perfectly allowed to know, without a doubt, that what you are going through is not fair. Not even fair for a single solitary second.

*Chapter Thirteen*

# PRESCRIPTIONS & PERSPECTIVES

My mother is beautiful - not regular people beautiful but movie star beautiful. Somehow she has been married twice, both times to men who showed less-than-leading-man kind of behavior. She and my father were married until I was about two at which time he had an affair and left her. However, my mother never spoke ill of him to me. She even invited him and his new wife to functions and into my life. I graduated high school with all three in tow. I graduated college and all three were there. I was married and all three sat on the front row. I love them all immensely and would have it no other way.

My dad, after 21 years of marriage, has since left my incredibly fantastic stepmother. However I celebrated this Mother's Day with both my mom and my step-mom for brunch. Remember, my step-mom is the woman my father originally left my mother to be with. I think it takes an amazing woman (or women in this case) to rise above circumstances and grow a relationship of respect and ultimately friendship.

One day, while catching some Oklahoma sunshine in the neighborhood pool, I asked my mom how she did it - how she managed in the beginning to be so civil; welcoming even. How did she maintain composure and class? How did she not transform her life into the soap opera her beauty was made for? It had to have been so difficult.

She admitted to being human and that it was difficult for a lot of years. She bluntly told me: "I had a decision to make. I could either choose to be angry and upset for the rest of my life or I could choose to deal with it and get on with my life. I choose, for your sake Kristine, more than mine, to deal."

She taught me that day, while lying in our bikinis, that no one else can make you happy. You choose to be happy or sad. You choose how you react to a situation and how you allow that situation to shape you. Your response is your decision. I am a different person because of that conversation and the pillar of strength my mother built.

Therefore, you need not look to a husband or best friend for comfort and hope. You need not even look in the direction of your mother. You must search yourself for the strength to be happy. Find the inner power that gives you comfort. When it comes to your emotional health and your personal fight for a family, you have a choice to make. Maybe your family doesn't look like you thought it would. Maybe you adopt. Maybe you end up with one child from Africa, one child from Okmulgee, Oklahoma and one from Russia. Still, that is the family God wants you to embrace. You are the only one that can choose. To deal or not to deal – that is the question.

Since everything health-related requires a prescription these days, I wanted to share with you the prescriptions in my cabinet. Perhaps so you can find your own self-inspired prescription for "dealing".

My personal prescription involves one or multiple doses of the following necessities:

*Anything chocolate*

*Long girlfriend talks in person (no phone, just eye-to-eye and usually on the floor)*

*Kitchen dancing with my husband when there is no music on*

*Watching my favorite old movies or any movie with my favorite few actors*

*Candlelit bubble baths*

*A good sweaty workout*

*An episode of America's Funniest Home Videos (using my DVR to fast forward as needed)*

*Couch napping*

*Sweet tea and the front porch*

*A long belly laugh that you feel in your abs the next day*

*A long cry that lets it all go*

*Reading a book next to the fire with our dogs nearby*

*A solid high five*

*A long walk at the lake (or anywhere really)*

*Deviled eggs*

*A chai latte and a biscotti (this is taken daily)*

This really is a non-ending list. One day a bubble bath will do the trick. The next day, I may need Shanghai Noon with Jackie Chan and Owen Wilson while eating chocolate and preparing for a couch sleep. The point is, I have learned what I need to bandage my pain. I have figured out what makes ME comfortable.

I can call my mom and, after telling me the needed words "just breathe," she will try to solve my problem by mapping out necessary steps toward the goal (there is no question why that woman is so successful in business). But, most of the time, that is not what I need. I need to comfort myself.

So, use this page to write your own prescription for comfort. Add to it as you think of new must-have happy makers. Maybe even rip it out and post it somewhere. I have found that when I am in a deep, dark, no-end-in-sight kind of sadness, sometimes I can't see my way out. This is when posting the prescription will pay off.

Just tell your husband to reference the prescription taped to the freezer, should he need to. And the truth is ladies, your hubby will probably know when to reference – am I right?

Hi, my name is _____

and this is my prescription for making myself happy. If you are not me and you are reading this, please feel free to do all you can to make me happy. I am not opposed to that one single bit!

1.

2.

3.

4.

5.

6.

7.

8.

9.

10.

Don't just turn the page. Really, get a pen and fill in the blanks. This is important and kind of fun.

Nothing I can write or say is going to give you 100% comfort and hope. I know and understand that better than anyone. In fact, you may have turned to this chapter and thought to yourself "this should be good." (Sarcasm, of course.) However, I hope you have a bit more optimism than that after reading the other chapters. The sting of the situation is still felt even through a good belly laugh or two.

When comfort and hope are in short supply, there is really only one place left to turn: God. Often you will find tenderness in prayer that cannot be found elsewhere. God knows your true emotion. He does not see your mask, He sees the real unaltered you – like it or not. Because He knows you so well, He also knows what you need and when. Our most difficult challenge is listening to Him. I am certainly a novice at this and pray often for help in hearing His "voice," but there are times when I am positive God is tenderly holding my hand.

*Journal Entry*
*The anniversary of another year of unsuccessful treatments. And we had just learned our first round of IVF did not work.*

*I took a walk. I went to the lake - my special place. There are walking trails in the woods with lengths of 3 or 6.5 miles. There is a dock and there are many great lake front places to sit. I did not want to walk long so I measured the circle drive around the park's parking area. It's .7 miles and I decided to walk it three times. On the third time I was feeling like there was no end to this emotional drain. That I was destined to pep talk myself every day into getting over this pain. So, I had a talk with God.*

*He and I tend to speak in songs and, at this point, two verses from different songs came to me. "Sometimes he calms the storms and sometimes he calms his child." Powerful! "And some things are the way they are and words just can't explain." (from Never Saw Blue Like That by Shawn Colvin).*

*(Soak those songs in for a moment. Get on Pandora, I-Tunes or Rhapsody Web sites and listen to the words.)*

*I walked to a part of the lake's shore where the land juts into the water a bit. A small peninsula by definition, I suppose. I stood there with my arms open wide, no one around, wind strongly blowing against my face. And I confessed out loud all my feelings to God. I have thought of them many times but never out loud into the wind. It was beautiful. Then I stood there listening with eyes closed to the waves, small, crashing against the rocks that lined my peninsula. I got down in a squat, put my hands in the water, asked for forgiveness and for God to treat this like a baptism. Then I rubbed my forehead with water the way you see on some movies.*

*I have trusted God for several years now but have never been baptized officially. I am scared of doing that in public even though part of its whole goal is a public profession of your faith in Christ as Savior. I passed out at my wedding. Can you imagine how much more important this is? I am scared the emotion would engulf me and I would drown.*

*My little peninsula baptism does not make me different, though I feel God being glad I did it just as an act of obedience and surrender to Him. I walked to finish that third lap and there you have it. The wind did not hit me as strongly. My thoughts were not on my dire situation but on the importance of teaching the Word and using my given skills. I thought maybe He is calming both the seas and His child if only mildly. He is God. He can do that.*

Talk about some much needed comfort. I was not any more hopeful as to the outcome of my situation, but I was not focused on it either. God knew that I would not suddenly forget my problems. He just found a way for me to redirect myself, if only for moments.

Changing your perspective is an amazing way of dealing with the world around you. I have found myself doing this in all kinds of situations, especially driving. When someone is tailgating me and then zooms past at an erratic rate, I have found that if I think to myself "he is getting to the hospital because his wife is in labor." This allows me not to toss him the bird. If someone is driving so slow I think "they are taking their new child home for the first time," or "this is that old person's last drive before he retires the keys." I find a great deal more patience for people in these scenarios.

Perspective is powerful. The more frequently you can adjust yours toward the positive, the more you are going to enjoy life – or at least tolerate it.

*Journal Entry*

> *I want to jump back to the last ten days. They have been wonderful. I am so thoroughly blessed in this life that I worry I will be disappointed in heaven.*
>
> *I have the most amazing husband who constantly impresses me. Matt believes an un-evaluated life is not worth living and he is always trying to improve himself in work, social situations, at home and with Christ. I have learned so very much from him lately.*
>
> *I have the best group of friends a girl could ask for. They are fun, exciting, always ready to laugh, cry or climb a tree. I have no doubt that in any kind of need I will have at least five amazing friends that will never turn me down. I am so rich in my friendships that I make Bill Gates look like a bum. My family, though thick in its abnormalities and dysfunctions, is supportive, loving and always by my side. I live in a wonderful community where I don't have to lock my home or car door and I got a note on my windshield when a man slid into my passenger side door during an ice storm. I have a wonderful church and pastor. My bed is comfortable. My heater works. My clothes are almost in style and I don't care very much one way or another. People like to spend time in my home and feel comfortable here. I have learned to sew enough to get by. My new cell phone requires that I type in all the phone numbers again and I got to realize how many people I love.*

*My shelves are full of books I read, loved and can't wait to share or can't wait to get started on again. My refrigerator is full of things that make me full. My dogs are handsome and almost well behaved. All my pens work. I have learned to use my husband's 3,000 button remote control for the television. I have been to Europe. All the people I know well are healthy.*

Even in the midst of pain, joyful days – even excessively joyful satisfied days – can come. Savor them. Soak them up. Slow down long enough to recognize and appreciate them! If you're thinking "yeah, but I don't have those relationships and that life and time to talk to the wind," then make those relationships, create the life you want and find the time for whatever helps you. Comfort and Hope - Make it. Create it. Find it.

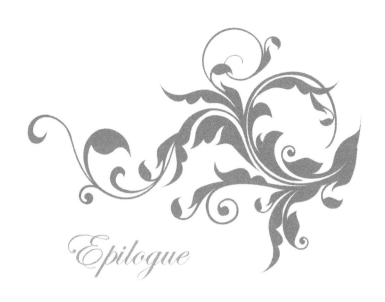

# WHAT DOES THIS DO TO YOUR BOOK?

*I* have heard this question a number of times in the last couple of months. What does THIS do to your book? My answer is easy... "nothing."

Let me explain.

As you saw in the Acknowledgments section of this book, one of the people to whom this book is dedicated is my beloved mother-in-law, Dana Waits. She is the kind of woman we all strive to be in so many ways. She gives full attention to others when they tell stories, remembers birthdays and baby names, says hello to people in the grocery store that she barely knows, hosts the company Christmas party, hugs tightly, knows her second cousins well and I could go on. She is true to the kind of woman God created and cherishes.

Unfortunately, I should say "was" this kind of woman. In December 2006, she was diagnosed with a rare and aggressive form of cancer called Inflammatory breast cancer. If you have not heard of it, I highly recommend you do some research. Mammograms don't pick it up and by the time it is discovered, it has usually spread through the lymph system and is throughout the body. This was the case with our Dana. She put up a valiant fight, never considering the end result of her cancer to be terminal. She only had positive things to say and never once used words of giving up. The outpouring of love from her family and friends was what, I believe, sustained her for a time.

She was taken from this earth and from our family in June 2007, less than six months from her diagnosis and less than two weeks from her only grand-baby's (our son Sam's) first birthday.

During those end days, I prayed fervently about her condition. I literally spent hours on my knees, which is not a position I have ever prayed in before. I rubbed her photograph telling God "please Lord, she deserves to stay."

One night, as things were eminent, I stood alone in her library sobbing and praying with an intensity that I have never known. This was more intense than all the fertility prayers I had ever prayed. If you have lost a loved one or have had the occasion to potentially lose a loved one, you know exactly what I am talking about. It is a mourning, hopeful, pleading prayer that exhausts every cell in your body.

During that time, I had a moment when I knew God was with me. I was begging God in a repetitive and almost chanting way "make a miracle, make a miracle, make a miracle, make a miracle." It was all I knew to say. Then it happened. A peace within in my soul that can only be created by our Savior came over me, changed my posture and closed my mouth. God told my heart "I already have." And that was it.

At the time I thought it meant either that Dana was going to pull off some kind of amazing healing or that the last few days of her lucidity had been that miracle.

Dana died. I do not blame God. I thank Him for the time we had, the influence she gave so many and the grace with which she was able to leave.

I was ill. I threw up all the time. I missed Dana in my soul and I thought for sure that this was the reason for my sickness. The day after she passed, I could not take the sickness any longer. I phoned the doctor and begged to come in. I needed something to make this better. No doctor could see me for several weeks.

My stepmother, Michele, was with us a lot during that time to help with Sam and all the unexpected meetings and such that happen at a time like that. Michele recommended I take a pregnancy test. I rolled my eyes, knowing pregnancy was impossible for us without medical intervention. However, after a few more fits of nausea, I gave in to her recommendation. At least I would be able to tell the doctor that is an item that has been checked off the list.

I bought a pregnancy test, peed on the stick and got the news. Positive.

Of course I did not believe it. So I phoned my local ObGyn and told them I had to come in immediately for blood work. It was 4:30 p.m. The lab personnel had gone for the day but if I wanted to pee on one of their sticks, I was welcome to do so. Matt and I packed up quickly and headed over. It was seconds after peeing that the nurse gave us the news – pregnant.

In the abandoned waiting room Matt and I cried and screamed. The nurses and office staff joined in. We told them that Dana had died only yesterday and that this was a pure blessing. More tears came.

I was 7 weeks and 3 days along. It had taken two rounds of IVF to get our first child and it had taken the death of one of my best friends – my mother-in-law – to get the other.

We announced the news to the family immediately. We were certain that Dana had gone straight to heaven, stamped her foot and said "God, I would really like more grandchildren." And so it was.

I do not question now what God meant when He said to my heart "I already have." The miracle He created was within me. Praise His mysterious ways.

So you see why I have been asked "What does this do to your book?" How can I continue to write a book about the I word and have conceived on my own, by accident no less?

That answer is easy. Just because my body figured it out this time does not mean that I did not experience every moment of the pains of infertility. This miracle, in fact, is proof of the inconsistency of fertility and the miracles that override science every day.

Katherine Dana Waits was born the following January. She has her Grammy's eyes, along with her name.

We still have four frozen eggs that we pay to store each month. Who knows what lies ahead?

All I know is that… you never know.

Keep your hope alive for tomorrow and be the person you want to be today.

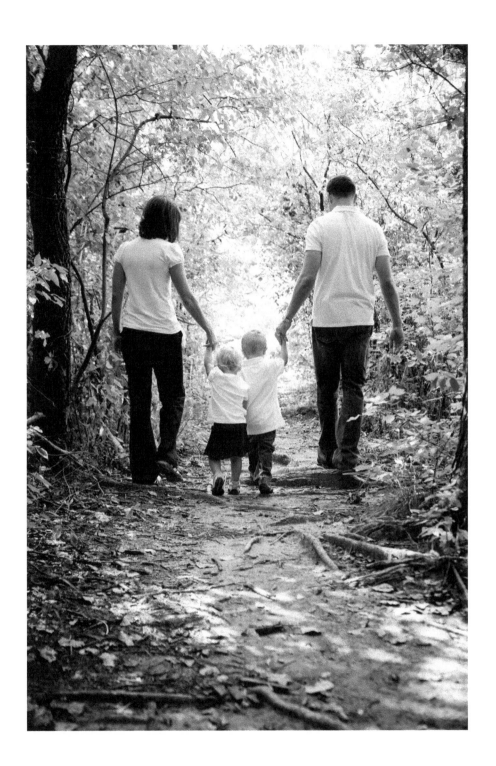

CPSIA information can be obtained
at www.ICGtesting.com
Printed in the USA
LVHW111526280219
609069LV00002B/367/P